CLEAN **REGIME**

CLEAN **REGIME**

A Health Coaching Guide to Achieving Vibrant Health

MICHAEL ESPINOLA

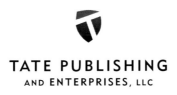

TATE PUBLISHING
AND **ENTERPRISES,** LLC

Published by Tate Publishing & Enterprises, LLC
127 E. Trade Center Terrace | Mustang, Oklahoma 73064 USA
1.888.361.9473 | www.tatepublishing.com

Tate Publishing is committed to excellence in the publishing industry. The company reflects the philosophy established by the founders, based on Psalm 68:11,

"The Lord gave the word and great was the company of those who published it."

Book design copyright © 2012 by Tate Publishing, LLC. All rights reserved.
Cover design by Rodrigo Adolfo
Interior design by Jomar Ouano

Published in the United States of America

ISBN: 978-1-62147-579-8
1. Health & Fitness / Healthy Living
2. Health & Fitness / Nutrition
12.10.04

Table of Contents

Disclaimer

The statements made here in this book have not been evaluated by the FDA and therefore are not meant to treat, cure, or prevent disease.

We have to say this because the FDA has not officially said that these concepts and statements are healthy or if they are safe. But you can decide for yourself under the liberty of freedom to choose what is right for you; however, *always* consult a licensed healthcare practitioner before you start any exercise, diet, or cleansing program of any kind. Any changes at all in your regimen should be made in a productive, informed manner, so if you are unsure, you should check with your doctor, again, *before* you take any new foods, herbs, plants, or supplements as well as any new drugs of any kind.

Preface

Are you sick and tired of being sick and tired? Are you fed up with feeling sluggish and ill? Are you someone who wants to be healthy and vibrant? Does the amount of disease in our world today make you uneasy to say the least? If you're like me and you want to feel a state of well-being and vitality and feel a need to stay healthy and young for life, but you are confused as to how to go about it, then you've come to the right place! With so much information out there about what is healthy and what isn't, it's not easy to figure out what to believe or which products contain truly healthy substances. It doesn't make sense that a consumer should be educated on the healthy characteristics of a food, drug, hygiene, or cleansing products by simply listening to the people who are creating and selling them with the use of commercials in the media. You should want to know for sure which substances will enhance our health and which substances either don't help at all, or worse, are actually causing damage instead of healing.

We have all heard by now that high fructose corn syrup and hydrogenated fats are bad for you, which I believe is true; however, the fact that someone knows these two pieces of information is far from having enough knowledge to be effective at preserving our health, which is becoming more and more obvious today. In this book you will learn how to make sense of the different claims and opinions of what is healthy and what isn't by learning how to decide this for yourself.

This book will discuss in length the most common food and cosmetic and cleansing products that we expose ourselves to daily, which are actually causing damage to our bodies right now. At the same time, I will discuss simple concepts that can be applied by the layperson at will, which will help you make the right decisions when choosing which of these types of products are safe to use or not. Internalizing this information will allow you to apply it in your life, which will help you to avoid becoming a victim of greedy and immoral business practices in order to live a fulfilling and healthy life.

Purpose

The purpose of this book is to share with you some information that was introduced to me over the past several years through observation, research, and implementation. This information has not only helped me achieve vibrant health but has turned back the clock of aging, making me look and feel decades younger (which people notice). It has allowed me to address my health issues in a more informed manner, discover what was causing them, make positive changes along with my doctor, and further reverse negative health ramifications, which were caused by the exposure to harmful chemicals. We do this first by removing the existing contaminations from our regimen and later preventing them from happening in the future. This process is achieved by first cleansing toxins from the body and further removing them from our regimen of food, hygiene, and cleansing products.

If not for a continuing enthusiasm of health concepts, this book may never have become a reality. This insatiable curiosity led to my enlightenment; these new eyes gave me the ability to develop the skills to achieve vibrant health, and now I wish to pass this information on to you. Because this experience was so eye opening, spiritually uplifting, and physically liberating, I have decided to make it my life's work to help as many people as possible by sharing this wonderful experience here in this book.

From the very beginning, I wanted to do something to help people. Later when I realized my passion for health and nutrition, I decided I would do something to help others with the same goals to get and stay healthy. And since I am so passionate about truth and justice as well, it seemed like the way to go. I wanted to do something about the lies being perpetuated by the corporate machine via the media, which are like a virus in the mind of man. I couldn't stand watching people become victims when I knew that there were ways to avoid becoming one.

It is not my intention for you to accept each and every word that I say without further investigation of your own. I do not expect you to agree with everything that I state in this book, but I do ask you to keep an open mind and take a look at some of the concepts presented here, because I believe if you do, you too will have the knowledge to make positive changes in all aspects of your life. No matter what your calling is, what your goals are, or what your profession is, having the ability to achieve success and be all you can be starts with vibrant health.

Without your health, you lack the foundation needed to achieve any successes in life. All too often today, even the brilliantly successful people are being struck down by disease in their prime. Staying healthy is a freedom included under the umbrella of liberty. I urge you to take control and responsibility for your own health. Be your own health advocate; communicate with and ask questions of your doctor, investigate different concepts of therapy and healing, and further be confident that you can make informed (with the help of a licensed health practitioner) decisions about your health. Don't forget to trust in the Creator and the tools that he has left for you, for it is the best way to become whole again and stay that way.

This book should be read from cover to cover, as all the chapters are equally important. The book has been outlined by breaking down each chapter with reference points for each specific topic being described. This will allow easy reference later as you try to research and apply some of these concepts into your regime.

Introduction: The Nation's Health

The condition of our nation's health is quite startling. Over 50 percent of the population is obese, and this number continues to rise despite the billions of dollars spent on "healthy" diet foods and programs. Not to mention the plethora of workout DVDs and pieces of exercise equipment being advertised and sold on TV every day. There are so many who are sick; it's all people talk about. Doctors and medicine everywhere I go, stories of doom and disease, infections and medications, conditions and disorders, therapy and rehabilitation, testing and diagnosis, worry and anxiety, surgery and infection, and on and on. This typically saddens and often annoys me when I hear this, knowing what I know. Maybe when you know, you'll be saddened too, and probably even a little angry.

The healthcare industry is booming, reporting record profits with more and more businesses opening every day. If you pay attention, you'll see a new commercial, building, doctor, technique, drug, drugstore, walk-in, hospital, or other business related to healthcare being implemented all too often. We are spending as much as 2.5-plus trillion dollars a year on "healthcare" and more every year. Outlooks on employment rank the medical industry with the highest salaries across the board, from surgeons to nurses, to medical sales and manufacturing, to investing and research.

But wait! If business is booming in the healthcare industry, doesn't that mean that more and more people are getting sick and staying that way? I'm pretty sure if the healthcare professionals and businesses are flourishing this would have to be true. It seems like there is a new disease being discovered every day, which leads to a new type of doctor, drug, machine, tool, surgical procedure, charity, and clinical study.

Marketing Tactics of Drug Companies

Watching any time of day, you'll see a new commercial or hear on the local news about a new breakthrough medical technology for an existing ailment, or worse yet, a new one (these new drug breakthrough reports always come out of the financial section of the news). Drug and other medical companies create de-sensitizing ideas in their advertisements that all can be well no matter what happens to you, based on the concept that the products and services that these companies *sell* will free you from any debilitating or terminal disease. Or that having and living with disease, and further managing it with their products is common and okay, when actually it is not okay, and certainly not how I wish to live. In reality the people involved with the manufacturing and marketing of these products and services are thinking how they are going to be rich when you become ill. They do this because they know we aren't aware of the truth, and so we believe their deception. Because many people are already ill, there will be many new customers for their new products and services.

I would like to state before we go any further that I believe in free enterprise and that not all successful and wealthy people are this way because they are bad or have earned an abundance of things in their lives from hurting others. There are elite groups of people, as well as everyday successful people, who help and benefit others (society). And there are elite people that live off the oppression and efforts of others who don't know any better. Unfortunately, there are more and more bloodsucking elite today as greed overtakes humanity. However, this doesn't have to be your reality as long as you don't let it!

These corrupt companies are using marketing tactics consisting of lies, guilt, half-truths, and fear to get you to run to your doctor for these medications, surgeries, and other "health" services they have to offer. I've seen commercials with a gurney following a man around, lurking in the background with scary music playing, and an announcer saying that if your blood work isn't perfect, you'd better take their drugs, or else you'll be on the gurney!

Another commercial portrays an older woman trying to share a very important life experience by taking her daughter to find a wedding dress. But alas, the whole experience was "ruined" because the mother had to go to the bathroom a couple of times during the event due to an overactive bladder or incontinence. The commercial totally ignores the causes of incontinence and how to cure it and instead convinces you that simply controlling the symptoms is tantamount.

Later, the commercial shows the "diseased" mother feeling guilty because she didn't take the drugs being advertised that would have ensured a great bonding experience with her daughter, with sad music playing in the background. All of a sudden, the sun comes out, the music changes to happy tones, and the mother and daughter emerge from under the sunrise holding one another's hands and smiling! Wow, that is awesome! What caused this major shift in atmosphere, you ask? Mom now takes the medication, so all is well. The mother and daughter have a perfectly fulfilling relationship because Mom no longer needs to go to the bathroom!

Health Professionals Who Care

Don't get the wrong idea; there is a place for drugs and surgeries, and there are many people in the healthcare industry who are true professionals who care, offer healing techniques, and choose to do the right things for the right reasons. There are health experts who know how to truly help people who are ill, and there are practitioners who are interested in facilitating cures because they care about other people. These healthcare professionals are out there, but there aren't many doctors thinking outside the box today. Sometimes this is true because they do not have the ability to act on their own beliefs and conscience due to their associations with these corrupt, greedy corporations that make the rules in medicine. Don't forget the golden rule: "He who has the gold makes all the rules!" So much damage happens to people from drugs, but it is always the doctors who are put to blame when things go wrong, that is if anyone gets blamed at all.

More People Sick Every Day

Despite the plethora of modern medicine available, the fact is more people are getting sick every day. It seems to be just getting worse. I don't recall when I was a child hearing about so many people getting cancer or having all these diseases we have today. Every now and then you would hear how someone distant from you—like a friend's uncle—has cancer, but now we all have someone close to us that has some kind of disease or illness that is *chronic* or *terminal* and must take medication for the rest of their lives in order to "be well" or even stay alive! And sadly, many more of us have lost loved ones to disease, either recently or in the past.

Wondering why there is so much drug use, I ask people about it and talk to others all the time who tell me that they *have* to take multiple prescriptions on a daily basis. One half is for their array of ailments, and the other half is to deal with the problems (side effects) that the first half causes. When I asked them why they feel they need to take so many pills, the typical answer from them is that their doctor *makes them* do it.

I don't doubt this is true, watching the commercials for pharmaceuticals made to save people from debilitating disease portrayed by doctors (actors in lab coats) doing just that, urging you to take this medication as it is their belief that this is the *only* way you'll get and stay healthy. Other commercials show actors portraying the actual patients, confessing how they made a huge mistake by not taking these medications in the past and as a result suffered some disaster with their health. But you don't have to learn the hard way if you just listen to them now, do the right thing, and take these medications. I often wonder if we ever ask ourselves the real causes of our health problems. Do these drugs actually offer a true cure, or do they merely hide the problem by masking it with symptom management? Worse yet, do they actually perpetuate deteriorating health? Doesn't it make sense that if we address only the symptoms that we are really only ignoring the causes?

Contamination: the Cause of Disease

Upon extensive research, internalization, and implementation of this information, it led to the ability to successfully improve my overall health. I have drawn the conclusion that the real cause of illness is that our bodies are contaminated and stressed, which has left us with a chronically suppressed immune system. It has left us with bodies that are dehydrated, bloated, overweight, hungry, tired, sick, diseased, stinky, with chronically suppressed immune systems leading to chronic conditions and depression. And if you've ever read or heard of the side effects caused by some of the drugs being used today, you'll realize that the result of using them only further suppresses your immune system, either by accident or on purpose.

Scenario: I go to the doctor because I'm a little stuffy due to seasonal allergies. He prescribes me a popular allergy medicine, which I take, despite the warnings of dangerous side effects. Months later I contract lymphoma! This is disheartening to me, as I can't help but think about this actually happening to real people—adults and children. Maybe when we see or hear about it on TV, all too often with a "no big deal" attitude being portrayed by actors, it allows us to be detached and desensitized from this reality. That is of course until we are forced to face the devastating reality of disease when we or our loved ones contract some type of illness.

I realize some of these side effects can be rare *and* that some people use some drugs with apparent successful evasion from negative side effects. But who would want to risk serious illness as a side effect simply to remedy the sniffles or itchy, watery eyes? The idea is ridiculous to me, especially when I know that there are other remedies, safer remedies to help deal with symptoms as well as address causes of seasonal allergies.

Yes, allergies are caused by an increase in histamine, but have we ever asked ourselves what causes us to have an unnatural increase of histamine when the items that we allergic to are typically harmless to the human body? This is the part that most people don't get; we forget to ask ourselves and our doctors why we have allergies.

Allergies are a dysfunction within the body, which means it shouldn't be that way; it is not normal. Yes these things that are going wrong with us, such as allergies, are becoming more and more common as more and more people live the same lifestyle, eat the same foods, have the same exposures, and because they watch the same TV, have the same mindset. All we do is manage the symptoms and never really work on why or how we get these bodily dysfunctions in the first place. Any disease, condition, health situation, or aggravation is not normal, and most likely can be avoided.

Steps must be taken to cleanse the body before it's too late; the longer the contamination exists in the body the more damage to the body's internal organs, the more damage to the organs the more dysfunction within the body's systems, the more dysfunction within the systems the more difficult it is for our bodies to heal themselves of these injuries, as well as the added challenges in fighting off infection.

Just like other living creatures in the world that must eat and breathe to stay alive, when *we* do these things, we expose ourselves to more contamination. More time equals more consumption; more consumption equals more exposure; more exposure equals more contamination. These components tied together show the compounding effect creating the idea that the longer we live and the higher on the food chain a body is (we are on the top), the more contaminated our bodies become. That is why it is so easy to hide the effects of chronic exposure of contaminants over time with the concept of aging. Yes, the food, drugs, and cosmetics that we use today can actually age you faster, even some of the so-called "anti-aging" serums and compounds.

The more contaminated our bodies are, the more damage and severe the resulting health problems are going to be. When we are young, our bodies are less contaminated, and, therefore, the effect of this contamination is minimal. As we get older and the years pass, our toxicity levels increase with every breath, bite, or drink, not to mention all the contaminants that we don't think about.

Because this is true, the effects of this contamination become more serious as we grow older because it builds up over time, which causes dysfunction in the actual cleansing process and general dysfunction. Unless your lifestyle can keep up with the mess—meaning you practice a clean regime. Therefore, the toxicity of the body is maintained at a healthy level. At the same time, it seems as if we are reaching higher levels of toxicity earlier than we did in the past; if more disease is the result of more contamination, it seems we have a lot more of it today than when I was a child. So it seems we are far more rapidly reaching old age on a level of contamination and health issues than we did in the past. Keep in mind I realize that there is always an exception to the rule, and you should too.

Side Effects of Prescription Medications

One reason that some people are more susceptible to having side effects and others not so much is due mainly to lifestyle, environment, and genetics (body chemistry). Another reason that some people are more susceptible to these ill effects is due to an existing suppressed immune system. What this means is that if your body is dysfunctional and sick when you begin taking drugs, you are more likely to experience problems than if you were well when you began. The safest way to avoid side effects from drugs is to be healthy before and while taking them! When your body's systems are functioning properly, this allows you to be able to deal with these unnatural chemicals in a more productive, functional manner. In other words, metabolize, neutralize, and eliminate these toxins from the body.

Taking drugs can be even more dangerous when you're sick then if you were healthy! It sounds strange, but it's true. The problem is none of us needs to take medicines when we are healthy. Being healthy negates the need for pharmaceuticals. Natural substances, when used in their pristine condition (especially plants and plant oils), have no serious side effects and are universal to all genetic variables in humans. More importantly they can and are used safely and beneficially, whether you are sick or not. Also there are very few and very mild ill effects when dealing with interactions between two or more natural substances meant for human consumption.

Drug Interaction Problems

Some drugs, when taken together or even by themselves, prohibit the use or consumption of basic fresh vegetables, due to the interaction between the drugs and the vitamins and minerals contained within the vegetables. When one uses truly all-natural compounds in their whole, original form, there are no interaction complications between them. These all-natural substances work together with each other and your body, not against it or despite it. The drug companies like to use that same language (that their products work with your body) when describing their drugs, but there is always an interaction and side effect warning included with their products, as they are always designed to perform a specific task, despite your body's cooperation.

Drugs Interacting with Chemical Contaminants

The next problem is, if these drugs are so dangerous to mix with chemical compounds such as vitamins, why they don't tell you to stay away from all other chemicals while you are taking this medication? This doesn't make sense. What about mixing blood pressure pills with preservatives? How about depression medication mixed with hydrogenated oils? Are you telling me that they took all this into consideration when discovering and disclosing the interaction warnings of their drugs?

I doubt it. It seems more likely it would be impossible to truly understand the ramifications of *all* the different possible interactions between all the different chemicals we expose ourselves to. Once again, this reinforces the concept of a truly all-natural way of life, being the safest plan. Besides, I think it's painfully obvious what happens when we mix many new chemical compounds together and then expose ourselves to them—*rare* and *new* diseases!

Some Drugs Can Prohibit the Consumption of Greens

My father has taken a particular prescription, among many, over the years, which prohibits him from eating any green vegetables, except of course for canned green beans. Not good! The only vegetable he will consume for the rest of his life is a highly processed, nutrient-stripped, contaminated, dead, gray, useless vegetable. The reason canned green beans are okay for him to mix with his medicine is because they are so devoid of nutrition, there are no vitamins to interact with the drug. This was disheartening to me because I made the realization that he will never be well if he cannot consume fresh, green, nutrient-rich produce, and as a result he will be doomed to remain ill.

Unnatural Does Not Work with Your Body

Consuming unnatural chemicals is very dangerous, as they are not designed to work *with* your body. They do not provide enhancement to the body's functions and were never intended to be in our bodies in the first place; no matter what the TV tells you. Companies need to add these chemicals to their drugs, food, and cosmetics in order to maximize profit. They will consistently defend this concept, saying that we will all starve and die if we don't use these chemical remedies. They will further contend that in small amounts they are okay for you.

The funny thing is, the latter is probably true. A healthy body given the right nutrition can handle a small amount of chemical contamination on occasion. The problem is almost every company in the food, cosmetic, drug, or household chemicals industry is adding that small amount of "stuff" to their products, again supposedly being safe in small doses. But by the end of the day, all those small doses of unnatural substances add up to a large dose of a toxic chemical cocktail, which our bodies are showing the effects of by contracting so many new diseases today.

Drug Companies Making New Drugs Often

Pharmaceutical corporations are so fixed on making new drugs no longer out of necessity but for nothing more than financial gain for themselves and their investors. So much so that they are desperate to come up with *any* compound that can do *anything* even remotely effective; so they can get a patent, get it approved, and get it sold.

In recent years, as an example of this, there have been new forms of birth control coming on the market, all of which were advertised on TV, only to see that they were more dangerous than the leading birth control at the time. ABC's *Nightline* investigated the claims being made by the producers of Yaz as an effective form of birth control with the added benefit of helping women with severe PMS, only to find out that the drug had never been proven to help with PMS, and further found to be responsible for more blood clotting and deaths than the leading birth control product (Chris Cuomo, 2011).

Why did we need new forms of birth control if the existing ones have been used successfully for years? Why do we need multiple forms of NSAID or other drugs if the one we currently have is working fine, and if they come out with a new one and it proves to be better and safer than the first, why would we want to take the original one? Are the drug companies asking you to decide what is best for you in the end? Are we supposed to be qualified to do this?

Let's face it; with the ridiculous amount of side-effect possibilities, some worse than the original disorder being treated, we have to ask ourselves: Are these drugs really effective at healing and curing disease? Or are these drugs really just ridiculous attempts at manipulating the body in some way, giving their creators the Gaul to claim a healing power and further allowing them to corner the market of whatever disease they have chosen to "battle"?

If I were the highly important officer or individual to decide whether a drug should be approved or not, I think I would have higher standards, not allowing so many dangers. The problem is a corrupt corporation doesn't care if its drug is dangerous or even if people die. It has only one agenda: to make as much profit as possible. That doesn't mean every individual involved with this process is downright evil, but some of these corporations as a whole *are*, with their soulless citizenship and liability to the shareholders, the bottom line *is* the bottom line.

I would also like to clarify now, before we go any further, that I believe in corporations and big business. I believe that these concepts have facilitated enormous achievements that otherwise couldn't have been procured, or at least not as easily by any individual or small group. It is not the system that is bad, it is the way greed manipulates and corrupts the system. As an investor myself, I completely believe in public trading and business ownership of all kinds, but I will not enter into any transaction that does not benefit *all* who are involved. Business ethics have been lost through greed. I am here to tell you that there is enough to go around. We need only look to see the abundance of wealth we all have at our disposal.

Oftentimes a drug will be approved only to find out after a few months and a few million prescriptions sold that it caused multiple injuries and fatalities and is later taken off the market. Any sales are better than no sales! It only takes a few months of heavy marketing and prescribing to make billions of dollars, regardless of whether a drug can do anything productive or even if it is safe. These concepts have nothing to do with why they are being produced, approved, prescribed, and sold. Sure these companies would love to produce their own compounds that will actually do exactly what they want it to, without side effects, but they know that it cannot be done. Why? It's because it has already been done by our Creator and Savior and, like the wheel, cannot be reinvented or improved on.

Drugs Can Be Helpful

There are times when drugs are necessary and *do* help people, but *any* remedy should *not* have to be used long term, as this is not a solution to the problem. These types of remedies should only be used as a last resort or when it is a life or death situation, especially if the consequences could be death. Life or death situations happen when we don't pay attention to our health. We let ourselves get really sick, and drugs are the only remedy left that will work (theoretically) because the body is so damaged. Another example would be when we get into an accident and our bodies have been so damaged that some functions have stopped and need to be supplemented somehow.

If the concept of "only as a last resort" was implemented by people in mainstream medicine or culture, it would annihilate the pharmaceutical companies, as well as the overall medical industry. Because this is true, the truths about disease and cures are continuously suppressed through marketing and deceptive commercialism.

Due to overuse of unnatural products and remedies, our bodies are overwhelmed by toxins. And as a result, we have no way to gauge which types of remedies (natural or not) are better and safer for ourselves. When someone is exposed to dangerous chemicals on a daily basis, which most of us are unless we know better, we have chronic health problems as a result. Only later when we do hear about the benefits of fish oil and decide to begin taking it, it is unlikely that this small change will make any significant difference in our health unless more exposure issues and cleansing techniques are dealt with and used. When this happens, it only reinforces the modern medical concepts that scare us into believing if we don't use conventional medicine, we're living in the dark ages and taking chances with our health, when the opposite is more truthful.

The concept of creating an unnatural cure is a fantasy and would put the maker of the cure eventually out of business, leaving no motivation to do so even if they could. If you think drug companies are trying to find real *cures* for diseases, you have been sadly misled. I don't know if you noticed, but it seems that there are drugs coming out all the time. There are still no cures provided by them. Even cancer survivors are not considered cured by the medical industry. Once you get diagnosed with cancer, you are a cancer patient for life! (If you don't believe me, try getting private health insurance with a history of cancer!) When you have success in healing from cancer, they say you are in remission of the disease but still have it.

A corporation that manufactures drugs spends a lot of money to develop new drugs to patent. If a corporation were to invent a cure for a disease, there may not be enough profit created by the sales of the drug to make it worthwhile (for) to invest the money on the research of the "cure" in the first place. Offering a cure means no repeat sales, which could deem the whole process not economically viable. This is where charities come into play. They ask us to help find a cure and use emotional motivation and guilt, portraying the suffering of these disease victims, which is sadly and inevitably taking place in reality, to motivate you to take a stand against these diseases by giving money to these research foundations.

There are charities after charities collecting funds under the guise of trying to find a cure for some of the most common diseases. Two problems: The causes are being ignored, and there were no cures ever found within a pill as of yet. According to my beliefs and knowledge, there never will be. As a contributor to these charities, we are helping facilitate the continued profiteering of these people by lowering the research and development (overhead) costs of producing these new drugs by way of giving them the funds to do it! They use our money to find out the truth of what works in nature, only to suppress this information and use it against you later.

As an investor in a corporation, you have a right to access the actual information being discovered by the research that you have funded. As a philanthropist to charities, you have no right to the information gathered by these researchers; you'll just have to hope they do the right thing with the information discovered, of which you have helped pay for.

I definitely want to help people in real need, but I have decided to give money to local charities where I can see the difference it makes. Another way to help victims of disease is to let them borrow your copy of this book and take any monies you can raise for their particular disease and give the funds directly to the them. You will be doing so much more with your contribution. Not to mention the best gift you can give anybody is a gift of yourself and your time, so take time to help others in need, especially the invalid.

However if you have a charity that you give to and are positive about the intentions of these people's use of these funds, then you should continue to give. There are still a certain number of charitable organizations that are aimed strictly at helping people, where most or all of the funds go to the actual cause.

What *Is* Actually Manmade?

Whether you realize it or not; man has not created anything, at least not anything tangible, from nothing. All we have been able to do is take what God has given us and use them to create new things from these basics. We take elements and compounds found in nature and manipulate them to our liking. We have discovered some of the mysterious world of sciences, but we are still far from having it all figured out, especially when it comes to the functionality of the body and overall health. Regrettably, we tend to have to learn the hard way by fumbling around trying to reinvent nature. I do believe God wants us to put together different types of substances and to use his tools and gifts that he has given us to better our lives and relationships, but there is no need for the basics like food and medicine to be recreated, as they already exist and have for as long as man has existed or even longer.

Most of the time when drugs are produced, it is done by finding something natural that works as a remedy for an ailment (through research), usually plants, and then trying to recreate it, so drug companies can make it their own. One example of this technique is Lipitor, a cholesterol lowering medication which came from a derivative of red rice yeast. Another example is the new, patented form of fish oil. Supplement companies saw the market for fish oil was booming. Lots of people were buying and taking it. The problem is, any old vitamin-supplement guy or whoever can produce and sell fish oil. They said, "Let's change it enough so we can patent it. Then we'll convince people that our 'pharmaceutical' version of this fish oil is superior to the other natural versions on the market, scaring people into purchasing only theirs, thus cornering the fish oil market." (I do not believe in the use of fish oil, as it is *not a whole food* supplement, has too much processing involved with procuring it, and it can oftentimes be contaminated.)

The corporation commences with the marketing campaign facilitated through advertisements or even breaking news stories on television. Here comes the actor in the lab coat saying how once again they were able to improve on nature by modifying it somehow, and theirs should be the only type used because it is somehow superior to all other natural or unmodified versions of fish oils out there. Why fix what already works? The answer is it's the only way to have exclusive rights and corner the market. (Fish oil is a very healthy substance when it is consumed in its natural state, found in small, oily fish like sardines and herring. It is this form of fish oil that I endorse the use of.)

The Body Is the Vehicle of the Soul

When you expose yourself to dangerous chemicals and later rely on more chemicals to try to heal yourself when your body finally breaks down, it is as if you have relinquished all your power and control to others. You have allowed secular medicine to become your light and salvation; however, it will never be. God's plan for us does not include us being sick, diseased invalids, who are unable to live our lives the way we want to. God is your father. He wants for you the same things you want for *your* children, to be safe and blissfully happy! Happiness starts with vibrant health. Your "car" must be functioning properly in order to win the race. The race is not against others; it is the race to your own bliss in life.

One must choose and implement the tools and techniques from the ancient world as well as new information about existing plants, foods, and techniques. I often wonder how we were able to survive millions of years of evolution without any manmade/altered chemicals. You might be thinking, "But the all-natural medicines from the past don't work, right? They couldn't. I've tried green complex; I've tried calcium supplements; I've tried natural remedies, and they don't work. If I don't feel any major reaction to the use of these products, then I don't feel like they are doing anything. When I take drugs I know it, because something happens right away, which I notice, oftentimes through the manifestation of unfavorable side effects!"

Natural remedies and medicines do not always act instantly like taking a drug because they are subtle, gentle, and designed to work with your body's systems. You might not necessarily notice the healing effects they provide right away. When you take patented chemicals such as drugs, things usually happen right away. For example: When you take blood pressure medication, usually within a week or two (sometimes even sooner), you should see a drop in blood pressure, along with some side effects like dry mouth and constipation. The problem is these drugs do not work with your body. They simply cause something supposedly favorable to happen, which appears as if they have helped. In reality you are not well, and you have not been cured; you are just under the influence of a drug.

This remedy is not a cure to me, and this fact is especially obvious because of the need to continue to take these drugs in order to maintain your healthy blood pressure, or whatever other bodily function you are trying to manipulate. In reality the drug is keeping your body's systems under *its* control, where the body is forced to do what the drug is telling it to do, instead of actually bringing down blood pressure on its own through symbiosis, balance, and harmony within the body (true healing). Instead, your body must relinquish its own control to the drugs, leaving your health and healing in the hands of the chemist.

Natural Works When You Go All Natural

Another reason all-natural remedies don't work for some people is because of the continued onslaught of toxins our bodies have to deal with every day. If your body's systems are currently not working properly, then a natural remedy that works with your body's systems will not be as effective initially because they require your body's functionality, as they work directly with them. In order for all-natural remedies to work for you, one must make a commitment to remove as much of the unnatural from their lifestyle as possible, especially while their bodies are showing signs of dysfunction, which is the key to prevention of disorder and injury within the body.

Nature works when you rely exclusively upon it. If you ignore all the warnings of the contaminations in your body and environment, and do not take steps to protect yourself from them, you will inevitably become toxically overwhelmed. Your body's systems will become so suppressed that it won't necessarily have the *ability* to heal itself with the use of natural substances.

This overwhelmingly toxic environment within the body today is caused by the lack of the basic tools (nutrition), which the body uses to keep itself clean; therefore, it doesn't have the ability to rebuild, heal, or repair itself. True of course, unless you just so happen to live accidently a perfectly contaminate-free lifestyle combined with a consistent diet of nutritious food, which rarely happens today in the United States and other developed civilizations. There are still plenty of indigenous groups of people around the world with little to no health problems throughout their population and lives, living as long if not longer than people within our more "advanced" societies without any disease.

Because the average person's lifestyle creates so much contamination in the body, it lends to the reason so many people have to use drugs. The same people who make all the medicinal compounds are the same people who make all the other chemicals we expose ourselves to: preservatives, food additives, pesticides, herbicides, rat poison, insecticide, artificial flavorings, artificial colorings, cancer-causing sulfates and parabens, and every other man-altered, manipulated compound or isotope. So you see, if you live your life surrounded by these dangerous compounds, which are manufactured by these chemical companies, you will be destined to need more and more of their patented compounds and chemicals in an attempt to stay well.

It's often said that people spend more money on their health in the last two years of their life than the total amount spent during the previous years they have lived. This is often true but does not and should not have to be. We need to be more health conscious while we are healthy, instead of waiting until we are very sick. Prevention is the key to staying healthy, and so we must be proactive.

Eating healthy is not cheap, but you get what you pay for. If you buy cheap, you get cheap. I think we all know that. The concept here is quality, not so much quantity; eating better quality food, but less of it, can cost about the same. Most of us overeat today anyway. If we used all the money we spend on fast food, convenience stores, and coffee shops, we would have plenty of money to buy organic and better quality foods. Ironically, we eat more because we are hungry, but we are hungry because our bodies, no matter how much crap we eat, don't get the nutrition they need, which would satisfy our hunger in the first place. Our bodies are also chronically dehydrated, which can lead to hunger cravings as well.

Digestive Problems Can Cause Sugar Cravings

A reason for being continuously hungry is after consuming dangerous substandard food for an extended period of time, our digestive systems begin to become overwhelmed and break down, making it impossible to digest the poor quality food that we continue to eat. As time goes on, this is exponentially more damaging to the body and the digestive system. After becoming impacted with putrefying fecal matter, the intestines can become infested with parasites, fungus, and yeast. These organisms release enzymes (as well as poop) that cause sugar cravings and further contaminate the body.

Another problem is most of us don't eat breakfast in the morning, and some of us don't even eat lunch. This puts our metabolism into survival mode by shutting it down in order to conserve as much energy as possible, later turning on the cravings for high-fat, sugar, and calorie junk foods, which get worse as the day progresses, especially if we continue this fasting.

Most of us eat 80 to 90 percent of the food we consume on a daily basis in the late evening and or at night. When we eat a whole days' worth of food at night before bed because now we are starving, we cannot expect our digestive systems, which are dysfunctional from this habit and further have been shut down all day from fasting to deal with this giant acidic mess by digesting and absorbing it efficiently somehow. We also have the bad habit of eating too close to bedtime, which can lead to more digestive issues like chronic heartburn (acid reflux disease) obesity, diarrhea, and constipation.

These bad habits can make it even harder to consume breakfast in the morning. This is because when you go to bed with a full stomach, your digestive system tries to go to rest too. When you wake up, oftentimes you'll still need to finish digesting the foods that were consumed the previous evening. This is typically why most people "can't" eat in the morning. This condition, combined with a lack of proper hydration, leads to putrefying food in the lower intestines, which leads to further contamination of the body.

We Must Break the Dysfunctional Cycles

This is what we call a circular trap: situation A causes condition B, and condition B is the reason for situation C, and situation C leads us back to condition A again. This cycle causes us not only to be sluggish and overweight but inevitably is the reason why we have a buildup of putrefying food in our intestines, perpetuating the overall contamination of the body. Processed, chemically laden, modified foods, undigested and putrefying in the intestines and colon can directly cause intestinal cancers, syndromes, and other disorders of the digestive system, as well as all types of other diseases and disorders. These conditions usually, directly or indirectly, cause disease with this type of environment within the intestines. Anything that goes in your mouth ends up in your bowels—smoking, pills, mouthwash, food additives, liquids, toothpaste, and so on.

This is also a major contributor to the reasons why we have junk food cravings continuously. Our bodies are so undernourished and our digestive systems so dysfunctional that processed foods containing easily absorbed, high-calorie, simple sugars and fats are the only foods our starving dysfunctional bodies crave or can absorb for that matter. This is because these types of food contain the quick calorie fix our body is in desperate need of; however, this quick fix comes with a price. Typically when consuming these highly processed foods, sugars, and fats, only part of the foods are being used by the body; the rest of it oftentimes goes unidentified as food by the body, unable to be digested and again wreaking havoc on the colon.

In this book you will learn that we become ill either by getting a bug-related infection, or we experience a breakdown of the body's systems. In either case, it's due to a suppressed immune system and overall dysfunction of the body's systems. Our immune systems are being suppressed by a buildup of toxins in the body, caused by contaminated food and a lack of nutrition, as these are directly related. Another way is through the interference of the electrical systems (EMF) of the body as well as stress, both of which are directly related, as stress begins in the "wiring" of the body and directly interferes with the body's electrical system, communications, and overall functionality.

Also you will learn that all illness, including mental, is caused by contamination first, usually starting in the intestines (colon), and spreads to rest of the body. You further will learn how to cleanse and rejuvenate the body and learn to use basic tools in order to measure the toxicity of the body. Using these tools you will have the ability to maintain proper chemical balance within the body and learn how to avoid recontamination of our bodies by identifying the causes of and how contamination happens in the first place.

This book will discuss how everyday items in our regime and lifestyle are contributing to the overall contamination in our bodies. It will identify basic body chemistry and how it applies to overall health and take a look at the electrical systems in the body as well. Describing how and what interferes with them and how to avoid (shield) these electromagnetic forces and further learning how to rebalance our electrical systems and also reduce, manage, and eliminate stress.

And you will do all of this in order to achieve and maintain vibrant health, true health, for a lifetime. You cannot truly be free and happy unless you achieve and maintain vibrant health. When you are truly healthy, you can begin to achieve your life's goals and dreams. A person can be all that he/she can be. I guarantee when you experience it for yourself, you'll never have it any other way!

My Experience

It was June of 2008; I was an average thirty-eight-year-old man, knocking on forty. It seems my health was fairly typical for someone my age. Upon going to the doctor, I found out that I had a few different disorders shown in my blood work. High blood pressure, high cholesterol, high triglycerides, and slightly elevated fasting blood glucose levels were some of the symptoms of dysfunction.

Further, beyond just my blood work, I also suffered from chronic joint and back pain. I would get sinus infections or sinusitis three to four times a year, which would require antibiotics. I also suffered from chronic fatigue syndrome, needing several coffees a day, and come to find out later, an overall pH level as low as 4.5 within the body environment. Not to mention all the typical health annoyances that most people experience all too often today, of which you see remedies for on the television daily. None of this seemed odd to me, as there were plenty of people that have these kinds of issues and worse all around me and on television.

At this point, the only pharmaceuticals I had taken were limited to some painkillers when I broke some ribs or some antibiotics used to battle infections. Naturally I had taken plenty of OTCs, such as cough medicine, pain relievers, or blood thinners like aspirin. But I had not graduated to blood pressure meds, cholesterol meds, or worse, as I didn't go to the doctor that often, and I felt I was too young to need those types of drugs. Typically the only time I would go to the doctor was when I needed antibiotics for my sinuses due to infection. Whenever I would go to the doctor as an adult, I would already be self-diagnosed successfully beforehand, which is another reason I wouldn't go to the doctor too often. The only problem was, now that I was getting older, would I be able to continue to self-diagnose and self-heal, allowing me to stay away from the doctor much longer?

I always considered myself a healthy individual, trying to eat right and work out regularly. Surely if I do what the doctors say, "diet and exercise," I will be healthy, right? I should be fine. I won't be one of those people who are overweight, unhealthy, sick, and diseased, needing to take drugs on a daily basis just to stay alive! That's not going to be me. (Recently I learned that a friend with three children, ages eight, ten, and twelve, discovered all his children had high blood pressure and cholesterol. As a result their doctor wants to put them on cholesterol meds, even though they are so young.)

Health Problems at a Young Age

Even as early as twenty-eight years of age, despite my efforts to stay healthy, I had high cholesterol and blood pressure! I thought to myself, *How can this be? I exercise regularly. I cook most of my meals, don't eat out too often, and I don't consume a lot of processed foods like frozen dinners or fast foods. Also, I take vitamins and other "healthy supplements" on a regular basis. I eat a lot of fruits and vegetables, and I don't smoke cigarettes. What did I do wrong?*

I did, however, eat highly processed foods a few times a week. I did eat foods with modified sugars and fats. I did eat foods that were exposed to dangerous chemicals during growth and production. I did use common hygiene products that contain dangerous chemicals. I did expose myself to toxic dyes and cleansing products through the exposure of household surfaces and clothing. I did take common OTC medications several times a year. I did receive vaccinations and booster shots. I did expose myself to dangerous chemicals at work. I did receive X-rays and other forms of radiation. I did have exposure to mercury and other "heavier" metals thorough dentistry and pollution, and I did not consume a healthy source of hydration on a consistent basis. Pondering all of this, I took some of these questions to my MD.

First I asked him why he thought I was getting repeated sinus infections, requiring antibiotics to get rid of several times a year. To which he responded it is because of my profession, and the resulting onsite job environment. Since I have to go into people's houses and businesses all the time, this exponentially increases my exposure to these microbes. He assured me that needing antibiotics a few times a year was not out of the ordinary. He then further reassured me that he also has clients that he puts on antibiotics all year round! Well that doesn't sound so bad then. Since I only need drugs now and then, it didn't seem so worrisome or unusual after all. *Everybody gets sick in the fall and wintertime. I'm not special.* So I left it at that.

Genetics: the Universal Scapegoat

Next was to talk about blood work. Okay *why*, Doc? Why was my blood pressure high? Why was my cholesterol high? Why were my triglycerides high? Why was my blood sugar elevating? Why, even when I am consciously taking steps based on all the clichés reinforced in me for years, *why* is my blood work out of whack? With all the exercise and physical activity, watching of the diet, eating of fruits and vegetables and not a lot of fast or processed foods, *why*? His response was that it has to be genetic and that I will probably need pharmaceuticals to get my blood work under control since diet and exercise didn't do it alone.

When I tried to explain to the doctor what I had been doing as far as diet and exercise and other healthy steps, he didn't seem to have any opinion or interest in these methods. If diet and exercise actually work at keeping a body healthy, than I must be doing something wrong, and I need more information; however, my doctor did not have any more information other than the same old cliché: diet and exercise. Since I had been exercising as a bodybuilder and a trainer, I figured I was pretty savvy with the art of conditioning, again reinforcing the concept that there has to be more to this diet side of things.

The reality is that my doctor probably thinks I'm just saying that I am trying to watch my diet and that I exercise regularly, but all the while I'm not really doing so. This inept attempt at, or fabrication of, proper and consistent exercise is usually the case with most people, not only because of laziness but because of ignorance of the proper methods used to diet and exercise effectively. However, I knew that I had been doing the work and had been for a lot longer than he had been instructing me to. I knew there had to be more to it.

So his answer was genetics, which obviously takes all liability away from everyone involved, giving me a feeling of it is not my fault and I can't do anything about it. This concept leaves us feeling powerless and more dependent upon pharmaceuticals. No matter how hard I try to stay healthy, I'm supposed to believe that 50, 60, 70 percent and higher of the health problems we suffer today are caused by genetics. Funny, we survived and continued to evolve over millions of years without drugs, but the reason I have health problems today is genetics. There must have been a tremendous amount of genetic mutation that took place for the worse all of a sudden in the twentieth century and today!

Genetics Do Play a Role in Health

Despite my skepticism of genetics being used as a scapegoat for the cause of diseases, I do believe that there is a certain amount of truth to the consideration of genetic conditions that can cause you to be *prone* to something, and even some physical mutations, but I believe without the proper catalyst, these disorders wouldn't necessarily manifest themselves. That's why genetics are a good indicator as to possible future health problems. But this doesn't mean a person will have these problems for sure, nor does it mean that if they do have any health issues that they were exclusively caused by genetics and not some chemically toxic catalyst combined with a genetic weakness.

One toxic contamination can cause a particular illness for one person based on their genetics but could have a completely different effect and cause a different health problem for someone else with a different genetic blueprint. Just as a toxin might severely injure one person but not hurt another individual at all. This doesn't mean we should only focus on trying to avoid the health problems that our parents and grandparents endured. We should always focus on protecting ourselves from all disease, as no one is immune to the immense possibilities of health problems, even those of us who try really hard at staying healthy. If you do have a disease, you need to focus not on your disease but, instead, only on your healing.

I also believe that there is a certain amount of genetic mutations that take place where birth with a deformation or disorder is caused completely and exclusively by natural forces. I believe that this does take place in nature as well; however, I highly doubt that these things happen anywhere near as often as they would like you to believe. We know that birth defects are caused usually by some kind of contamination during fetal development. Studies have been done proving alcohol, cigarettes, drugs, and pharmaceuticals can cause birth defects. With the existence of so many of toxins everywhere in our environment and regime, it makes more sense that *we* cause most of the health problems compared to our genetic heritage or nature itself.

Free Medicine, Insurance, and *Lies*

So it seemed I'd be destined to be another disease-ridden person, who would have to spend the rest of my days being "under the influence" of prescription drugs, worried about filling my scripts, battling side effects with more scripts only to have declining health anyway. That's great! Looks like I'll have to get a degree in Medicaid so I can keep up with the enigma that is the US Medicare program now that I'll be taking part in those blessed "healthy" governmental administrations. "Don't worry, we make it easy," said the doctor. "The government will provide you with insurance if you can't afford it! We can give you discounted medicines and free trials when they are available. We don't even have to see you every time you need to refill your scripts. We can mail them to you so you won't even have to leave your house!"

Wow! These people really care about my well-being to go to all this trouble for little old me! I feel empowered and liberated. I feel like I don't have to worry about this stuff at all. My doctor, the government, and the pharmaceutical companies have taken care of everything for me, and all I need do is rely on them and do what they say, and I'll be fine! Sounds good! Almost too good. Free drugs and free healthcare? This doesn't sound right to me and cannot be the answer.

How can this stuff be free when these companies are boosting record profits continuously, and more people are getting involved and making more money? The reality is that it is not free. The healthcare system is set up to control us and to fleece us of our power and money directly from our pockets as well as indirectly through government programs meant supposedly to help us, when in reality these programs oftentimes are just more scams put in place by corrupt politicians and big business to get as much money from the "till" as possible for the people who have the power to do so. When you look at it in this way, it doesn't sound so empowering and liberating. And I'm not too excited about the proposition.

Drugs Do Not Provide a Cure

This is no solution to me. If I have a health problem, I want a real solution! And a solution to me in this case means a solution to the problem or a cure. I want a cure! I want to be made whole again! I thought to myself, *There has got to be another way!* It seems to me that the problem is that the real causes are not being identified, or worse yet, are being concealed. But why can't anyone tell me what these causes are, except for the basics like don't smoke cigarettes, don't eat too much fried food, don't eat too much fast food, don't drink too much soda, and all the other clichés in the book? I'm following all that, but nothing is changing. I still have blood work issues. I still have chronic conditions.

There has to be a logical explanation for this, something other than putting the blame on God or my genetic heritage. The problem was even though I didn't smoke, and I didn't eat too much processed food, I was still being exposed to all kinds of contaminants and carcinogens that weren't so obvious to me or anyone I knew for that matter, at least not right away.

The Book That Started It All

In 2008, I was given a gift. This gift was a book called *Natural Cures "They" Don't Want You to Know About*, written by a fellow named Kevin Trudeau. I had seen the commercial for the book on a local TV network and was intrigued by the title. So I bought it.

This same TV network had been on the air for years and always had some kind of self-help book or program, or a new, all-natural health product like kelp or green complex supplements, some of which I had purchased in the past because they sounded really good and made sense in how they worked. Trouble was, even though I had tried some of these products in the past, they didn't seem to make any significant changes to my health, which baffled me. There had to be some truth to this all-natural concept, but why, even though I had tried some of these all-natural products in the past, was my blood work still messed up? There had to be more to this. These products must work; they just need to be used properly. I thought to myself, *Maybe I'm doing something wrong.*

As an adult, I would often get most of my information from the TV, watching all kinds of programs on educational topics, science being my favorite. Now I said that I had received the book as a gift, and when it arrived, it did not make it to the bookshelf, as I was eager to find out the truth about how to cure my health problems. Needless to say, the awakening created a renewed interest in books and learning for me. I knew deep down inside that there had to be a way to reverse health problems, cure diseases, and become well again. I began to read the book on a Wednesday, and by Friday morning, I was making a commitment to changes in my regime, which I implemented that weekend!

Come to find out, the things that are causing disease and dysfunction in our lives today are right in front of our faces. Not only are the causes suddenly so obvious, but it was made clear that there are natural cures for what ails us. So if you find yourself sick, investigate and realize that there are alternative ways to true healing as well as additional therapies, which will greatly increase your chances of getting better, other than *only* through the use of surgery and pharmaceuticals.

More importantly I discovered that the way to avoid and/or address health problems is not to *add* more unnatural substances and chemicals to the mix but instead to omit some of these things that we are being exposed to on a daily basis. I found out that the health deficiencies that we suffer today are directly caused by the food we eat, beverages we drink, cleansers and hygiene products that we use, and pollution and other unnatural chemicals we expose ourselves to every day.

Everyday Items Causing Health Problems

I found it hard to believe, as do many others, that harmful products can be sold on a regular basis under the guise that they are healthy, good for us, and/or safe. As I read on, I was informed of many different known carcinogens that existed in the formulas of several of my hygiene products. There are sulfate and parabens contained within them that are, in fact, two known types of carcinogens found in many different hygiene products including toothpaste, bar soap, body wash, shampoo, conditioner, and moisturizers. These are two of the most common types of carcinogens, but there are many others as well as new ones every day.

Hearing this information, needless to say, was alarming. So I put the book down, went to the bathroom, and started to read the ingredients in all the different products that I use daily for hygiene health, only to realize that they, in fact, did contain these sulfates and parabens. *I can't believe it. There's no way that that this sulfate stuff is a carcinogen*, I thought to myself. If it was, this stuff would never be in these health products.

My next move was to go onto the Internet and search for information on these chemicals to see if they are actually carcinogens, only to find it was true. Sodium laurel sulfate is a well-known carcinogen. This was just one example of the use of a toxic substance in a product sold as a "healthy" one. Besides the sulfate products, my toothpaste, which is supposed to contribute to my oral hygiene, also contains fluoride, preservatives, modified sugars, and other unnatural chemicals.

The Big Question Answered

Well, that answers the question of why everybody is sick; or it's certainly a logical indicator! This is when I began to realize that the causes of our health problems today are being ignored, and worse yet, suppressed. It suddenly seems so obvious to me, yet I had lived thirty-eight years completely oblivious to these facts. Sure I have heard about preservatives, food coloring, and other basics that were harmful in food source. But I never dreamed that just about everything that I exposed myself to every day was contaminating my body, which was further leading to dysfunction and injury.

Okay, sounds like we're getting somewhere here. The problem remains: How do we know what is dangerous and what isn't? Does this mean I have to become a chemist and get a PhD in order to figure out what I need to stay away from versus what's safe? It doesn't seem right that the average person would have to know such things. This made me realize that I was going to have to become more aware, in order to avoid becoming victimized by evil and greed.

The Commitment of a Lifetime

So by the time I finished the book or even a little before, I had made a self-commitment to eat nothing but organic food from then on. I had no problem with this, as I am a "health nut" and have been for a long time. Not to mention this new type of food tasted so much better, which created a new love for food and cooking within me. I continued the thought process to include all of the cleansers I use in the house to all the cleansers I use on myself and my clothes, as well.

When Saturday morning arrived, I gathered all the food from the cabinets and refrigerator and packed them into my spare grocery bags. Continuing this enthusiastic purge of unnatural chemicals from the dwelling, I then proceeded to pack up all the cleansers in the house—dishwashing detergent, laundry detergent, spray cleaners, and any other unnatural cleansers I could find. Next, I gathered up all the medications, whether it was an OTC or a prescription drug. I then gave or threw away all of these items and then headed to the health food store.

Upon arrival, I couldn't believe how much all-natural and organic food that was available! I was a kid in a candy store, only the store was full of healthy candy! I purchased some all-natural plant-based household cleansers for cleaning not only the house but my clothes and dishes. Next was to find all-natural choices for hygiene like toothpaste, soap, shampoo, conditioner, and so on. It was all right there at the store, just like the book said. So began my journey to vibrant health.

Besides making sure that I had a handle on all of the things that I could control, what about all the stuff I have already been exposed to over the years starting at birth? What about any chemicals that could be trapped in our bodies right now, wreaking havoc? What do we do about them? What about all the future contaminations that we can't control? The answer to these questions is to *cleanse* the body now and regularly. (We will talk more about the specifics of detoxification later in the book.)

Clean House!

We said step one is to cleanup or cleanse the body, which will allow you to cool down and relax in order to realize a state of well-being. After your cleansing is complete, the body's organs and systems are going to begin to function more efficiently and harmoniously. This leads to the body recapturing its self-healing talents that it was born with, and further, it will begin repairing itself. This will give us a fresh start on our journey.

Next is to keep it clean by keeping and maintaining a clean regime and by cleansing your body once a year because of continued environmental exposure that you can't necessarily control, not to mention the unknowns. If you do not practice a clean regime on a regular basis yourself, you may want to cleanse your body several times a year in order to effectively keep your body in the best possible condition.

Once you have cleansed your body, it will begin to function properly again, and then it can begin to repair and heal itself, assuming that you continue to keep it clean. Yes, I said heal itself. You are the only one who heals you. Doctors do not heal, and surgeons do not heal; they only help facilitate healing. What this means is *you* are the most integral part of getting and staying healthy.

Physically Liberating and Spiritually Uplifting

I began my detoxification program that consisted of all kinds of clean, alkaline, ionic mineral water. I consumed tons of organic, alkalizing foods as well as plenty of whole food and herbal supplements. I addressed cleansing the colon, pancreas, liver, kidneys, gallbladder, bladder, lymphatic system, and blood, all done simultaneously without any special equipment or inventions. Within a week or two, I felt so much better and younger, with a renewed energy and vibrancy that I would look forward to each day as my cleansing continued.

We said that natural remedies don't react as fast as drugs when used to remedy chronic conditions or ailments, but I was able to feel better almost instantly. Despite this fact, my blood work was not perfect right away; it was not until after a few months of natural remedies and renewed functionality, in order to actually heal the damage that had taken place, before I saw results. In my case, I used cinnamon, which was used to lower my fasting glucose levels, combined with fish oil to battle high blood pressure. These remedies were prescribed by my N.D., and I believe that these natural remedies worked at helping to heal my physical issues, but I also believe that the removal of unnatural toxins from my regime and body, combined with feeling very healthy and vibrant, really made the difference in my overall healing.

Within a week or two, I felt like I was fifteen years younger. I had energy like I couldn't remember having as a youth! My skin was better, my hair was better, and I felt great! My joints didn't ache, and I wasn't tired. At this point, I was excited to have my blood checked again to see where I stood, as it had been a year or so since I had it checked. Since it had only been a short time since I started cleansing, the results were only a tiny bit better than they had been the last few times I checked, but I wasn't discouraged because I knew it would take some more time for the repairs to take place. I felt so good and so young; there was no way I was stopping now!

Hard-to-Believe Truths

Months went by and I was so excited about how good I felt that I wanted to share my experience with everyone. The more I talked to people about these concepts, the more I noticed that people (as I hadn't) didn't believe that food, cosmetics, and cleansers could actually harm them. They would often get overwhelmed and upset with me as I would share this information. This was mind-blowing to me because I felt like I was giving them invaluable information with no personal agenda or motive, other than to help, as I do not charge for health advice.

Oddly enough it seems people trust more in the guy selling them something with a clear motive to lie than a person discrediting these criminals with no motive to deceive them at all. They would react to my presentation of these concepts by arguing with me using the arsenal of information handed down to them by the deceitful profiteers through the TV medium. Using this information, people always have a contrary version of my information, defending the companies that make the products that they buy mostly because they use these products every day and don't want to accept the overwhelming idea that these products might be dangerous; nor do they want to accept the possibility that they have been duped, which causes an emotional confrontation and keeps them in denial. Anyway, this was not going to discourage me, as I know these healthy concepts work, because I feel great.

Six months into my clean regime program, I decided to go back to the doctors and have my blood checked. This time my blood work came back nearly perfect. I couldn't believe the improvement that had taken place in such a short time! And I hadn't taken one pill! Besides my blood work being almost perfect, my chronic joint pain was gone. This doesn't mean I never have an achy joint or other discomfort from time to time, but it means I do not have chronic joint conditions any longer. And if I do get body or joint aches, it usually lasts only the day, as a good night's rest and a nutritious meal work wonders.

Even more unbelievable was when the flu season hit; for the first time in my life I did not get sick. I'm sure that I was exposed to cold and flu microbes, but I did not get an infection as I did several times a year every year in the past. There were no more occasions where I needed bed rest or medicine of any kind due to being sick. My ND didn't seem surprised by this miraculous turn around in health, but my MD could not believe it! He said, "Hey, whatever you're doing, keep it up!" It was the best advice I had ever gotten from this doctor before. Too bad I had to figure it out on my own.

The problem is, the average doctor is just like you and me. They are regular people who aren't trained in the art of staying healthy. They are trained by the same people who make the laws and rules of medicine. They are educated in the latest technologies of disease maintenance and trained only to be disease experts, and not health experts. That's why doctors get sick; they get cancer, they smoke cigarettes, are obese, have diabetes, and "need" to take medicine like the rest of us. They are trained in damage control and symptom maintenance. Once they figure out what disease you have, based on the symptoms, they refer to the chemist to find out which of their products to prescribe you for your disease or condition.

This doesn't sound so God-like to me. Conventional medicine does not seem to offer any cures or any long-lasting health benefits. Even when you're going for a checkup, it seems as if they're just looking for problems, not unlike a dishonorable mechanic looking for things to fix that aren't really broken under your car. I constantly hear from medical supply companies at home on the phone. They are calling hoping to God someone in the house has diabetes or another disease and is in need of some supplies so they can make a sale. They usually hang up on me when they find out we don't need any.

Most people don't make appointments with their general practitioner to sit down and discuss ways that they can stay healthy and not become diseased or sick. That is why it is important to choose a doctor who really understands how to achieve and maintain vibrant health. Typically these types of doctors and health experts exist mostly in the homeopathic or holistic worlds of medicine, although more doctors of all kinds are becoming more aware of these facts.

The Simple Answers

So that's it! It so simple! Exposing ourselves to chemical compounds, elements, and/or isotopes that were not found in our natural regime or nature itself during our development through evolution are potentially hazardous to our health. These exposures are what cause most of the nation's health problems. Wow! Who thought it would be so obvious? I wanted to know more!

Here Are Some Other Things I Had to Consider Changing in My Regime

Cookware: Teflon

Plastics BPA

Aluminum Wraps

Paper products: chlorinated bath tissue, coffee filters, paper plates, and towels

Microwaves: release toxins from plastics and destroy quality foods

Stretching: Yoga-stress and EMF

Fluorescent lights: suppress the immune system EMF

Water for drinking and cleansing the body

EMF shielding from HDTVs, cellular devices, satellite signals, routers (hot spots), and other wireless devices, as well as machinery

Cavity fillings: contain mercury

Clothes: come new, laden with chemicals

Dentistry: fluoride and other chemicals

Air pollution: in the house, filters, plants

Wine: contains sulfites

Food origin: freshness

Stress: management techniques

Self-Motivation: staying focused

Sweets: even organic sugar is bad when overused

Fats: even organic good fats are bad if too much is eaten, worse is the modified fats as they are dangerous to the liver

Doctor: finding the right one to help

Environmental contaminations: air quality

Chemicals being used at work, "dust" Mycotoxin (mold), nearby industry

Immunization: mercury, aluminum, and formaldehyde

pH: Potential of Hydrogen

If you've ever taken a chemistry class; maintained the water in a fish tank, hot tub, or swimming pool, then you have probably heard of the term *pH*. What this literally stands for is "the potential for hydrogen" or "per hydrogen." Any body of water or water-based solution, whether it's a lake or a glass, has a pH reading. This measurement of pH has a scale from 0.00001 to 14. A reading of 0.00001 to 6.9999 finds you in the acidic range of the spectrum. A reading of 7.0 is smack-dab in the middle and leaves you completely neutral, where the acidic elements and alkaline elements are in balance. As such, a reading from 7.00001 to 14 will put you in the alkaline or base ranges.

Measuring Contamination in the Body

The next question I had was how do I know when I have effectively cleansed my body? How do I know if my body is still contaminated? Well, I found out that this is simple science as well. Your body is made of all kinds of elements and compounds; these elements and compounds are either acidic or alkaline. Just like in all aspects of life, we would like to achieve and maintain balance; likewise, our bodies want to achieve and maintain chemical and electrical balance. The chemical balance is represented to us through the measurement of the pH of your body environment. Your body, like I said, wants to maintain balance. This means on the pH scale that your bodily fluids want to be neutral or slightly alkaline. The problem is that most contaminants, pollutions, manmade chemicals, and life's stresses have an opposing acidic effect on the body. This is a major part of the problem with keeping our bodies in balance.

Everywhere I went I would talk about pH and try to get everyone to test their pH levels. Carrying pH strips with me at all times, I would test the pH of different water sources and other beverages as well. I spoke about how acidic, chemically laden drinks cannot promote balance or alkalinity but instead actually cause the body to become more acidic. Lots of people would seem very interested, asking many questions, and some others have even made major changes in lifestyle choices based on these concepts. Seeing this encouraged me to continue to share this valuable information with everyone I met.

Chemistry of Water

Water, unless it is distilled or contaminated, typically will be in solution of trace elements. Healthy water, for example, would contain your alkaline elements like calcium, potassium, sodium, magnesium, and so on, also trace amounts of other less favorable ones. When a solution has an acidic reading, it simply means that there are a greater number of acidic elements than alkaline elements. Likewise, an alkaline reading denotes that there are more alkaline elements than there are acidic. It is this alkalinity that is important to vibrant health, as the alkaline elements are the elements that help neutralize the acids and raise the pH in our bodies, which will help us achieve chemical balance within our body environments.

As you move from one whole number to the next, it's like moving at multiples of ten, where a pH of four is ten times more acidic than a reading of five, and 100 times more acidic than a reading of six. Within the acid ranges 0.1 to 6.99, the lower the number, the more acidic the solution is. And for the alkaline ranges 7.1 to 14, the higher the number, the more alkaline the solution is. An example might be that some intestinal juices can be as low as a pH of 2, where orange juice has a pH of about 6.5, and blood a reading of around 7.38.

I said that all water-based solutions have a pH reading, correct? Well, what do we know about the chemical makeup of the human body? It's made predominantly of water, correct? So as this is true, the body must have an overall pH reading for "its" solution of water.

Of course we realize, due to the need to digest food, that some of the fluids within the human body are acidic, right? We've all heard of heartburn from stomach acid. At the same time scientists, doctors, and maybe even you know that human blood is always slightly alkaline (7.35 to 7.43), or the person would suffer from acedemia (acidosis of the blood) and could go into a coma and or die. As this is true, so is it true that the most basic fluids within the body should also be as close to neutral or even slightly alkaline as well.

Organs Forced to Bathe in Acids

The organs and the individual cells of the body do not like to bathe in acids. Even your stomach uses sodium bi-carbonate to protect itself from its own acidic digestive fluids. The intestines, both small and large, sustain damage when the pH is not correct for an extended period of time. Things like Chrohn's disease, diverticulitis, IBS, and other digestive disorders are potentially caused by a consistent imbalance of pH levels (which simply represents the amount of contamination from toxins). This type of environment causes mayhem in the body and sets the body up for dysfunction. Some scientists think that this basic concept of pH balance and over acidity in the body is the root of all disease, as well as the way to achieving optimal health. I do as well.

How Does the Body Deal with Acids?

Because the body does not like to be acidic, it will do whatever it takes to achieve balance between these different types of elements. This balance is represented by the pH of our body's intra-cellular fluids. The body would ideally like to remain as close to a balanced range as possible (seven on the pH scale) or even *slightly* alkaline. The body does this under normal circumstances by utilizing its mineral stores to help neutralize the acidic waste within by the body. Once the waste has been neutralized, it can then be placed into the bloodstream to be eliminated by the kidneys. If the body were to dump acids directly into the blood *before* they are neutralized, this would lower the pH of the blood too rapidly, and you would again suffer from acedemia. This is why acids must be neutralized or made alkaline, first, before they can be eliminated from the body.

Problems with Nutrition Deficiencies

When we talk about nutrition, we are referring to the nutrients found within our food. Some of the common nutrients that most of us are familiar with are fats, proteins, carbohydrates, and calories. Some of us might think of vitamins and minerals when we are referring to nutrients. Different nutrients serve different purposes. For example, carbohydrates are to give us energy, be it a complex carbohydrate or simple sugar, it is the same; the difference is really only in the way we digest these carbohydrates. Complex carbohydrates take longer to digest, where simple sugars are already broken down and are readily absorbed by the body.

This is good for quick energy, but it is also a problem. By consuming too much sugar or simple carbohydrates of any kind (including organic ones), it will cause your blood sugar to spike, which causes stress on the pancreas and added acidity in the body. Proteins are required primarily because we rebuild cellular tissue on a regular basis. Therefore protein is used primarily for the production of cells and other types of hormones, enzymes, and tissues. But proteins are made of amino acids; this is why the consumption and synthesizing of proteins leave an acidic waste behind. (This doesn't mean that eating protein is bad, it just means that a healthy person is going to consume as much or more alkalizing foods then he does acidifying ones.)

Vitamins and minerals are the stuff that the body uses for cleansing and system operations. Minerals primarily are used to alkalize the acidic waste produced naturally and unnaturally in the body, as well as the conveyance of energy through the body, whether it's power for muscles or information being transmitted between neurons. Because today we have so many more sources of acids getting into the body, we would need to consume more nutrients in order to keep up with the added acidic wastes that need neutralization. The problem is that the foods we eat not only have fewer nutrients but contain more acidic elements as a result of processing and other unhealthy food production practices. This has led to the overwhelming unhealthy condition our bodies are struggling with today.

Besides the huge number of reasons our bodies become acidic now compared to 100 years ago, the extra nutrients that are needed to remedy the over acidity problems in our bodies are not provided by the foods available today. In fact, more often the exact opposite is true. Most of the food consumed today is more acidifying than it is alkalizing, leaving us with low or depleted mineral stores and an inability to neutralize acidic waste from the body. Consequently, the body ends up with a buildup of these acid wastes and ultimately in a state of over acidity whether it likes it or not, and it doesn't.

If there is a deficiency of minerals within the body, it will be unable to neutralize these acids for safe removal. When the body begins to realize that it doesn't have the mineral stores necessary to achieve the neutralization of this acidic waste (so it can be safely removed), it has a few emergency procedures that it can implement in order to protect the precious organs from this toxic, acidic mess.

Osteoporosis: Bone and Joint Loss

One way the body protects itself is to begin to rob the number-one, most abundant alkaline element in the body from the body, which is calcium. Since calcium is an alkaline element, when added to an acidic solution, it will raise the pH of said solution. Or in this case, neutralizing or alkalizing the solution of wastewater within the body. Hmm…rob calcium, isn't that bad? Yes, it is! It's called bone loss, or in the medical world, it is known as osteoporosis! This neutralizing technique also causes cartilage and joint loss (arthritis and calcium deposits).

Calcium is used as an acid neutralizer in other applications such as water-neutralizing filter systems for the home or industry. So you're thinking, *Oh, so I should take a calcium supplement then, right?* Not necessarily. Some calcium supplements cannot even be absorbed by the body due to the carrier or chemical "cohort," if you will. For example calcium carbonate (chalk) cannot be absorbed by the body and can only perform in the digestive tract as that is where it was placed; however, calcium citrate can be used by the body and is fully absorbed.

There is some argument about needing the presence of vitamin D in order to achieve full absorption of any calcium supplement. This is why I have come to the conclusion that a whole food supplement is always the best way to go. If it contains calcium, then by the laws of nature it will contain the exact recipe of cofactors necessary for the body to make full and proper use of the calcium and other nutrients contained within.

We have a drilled well that provides us with our domestic water for our home. This water straight out of the ground has a pH level of 6.3 -6.4, which is considered caustic. If we were to shower in this water, our skin would become very dry and itchy. If we were to drink it, we would be drastically adding to our acidity level, which is quite the opposite of what should happen, as water should be the primary tool for alkalizing the body. Acidic water will never be able to do this. A pure, natural form of spring water is always alkaline; this is why consuming clean, alkaline water will bring balance to the chemistry of the body when consumed on a regular basis. This doesn't mean if the bottled water has a label that says it is natural spring water that it is a healthy form of water.

With the use of a calcium-based neutralizer (filter), our water at home comes out the faucet about neutral. I can base the need to replace the calcium in the filter on how dry my hair and skin is from the shower. Also, I have copper water piping in my home. Acids break down the copper, leaving blue and green stains on the plumbing fixtures as well. If you have copper water pipes in your house and you see blue and or green stains in your shower or on other plumbing fixtures, it means that you have acidic water coming from your tap. If you live in a newer home, you most likely have plastic water pipe, which doesn't so easily indicate the presence of acidic water, and therefore you should have it checked.

Body Fat Being Used as an Acid Buffer

Another way the body deals with an overabundance of acids within, again as an emergency method due to a lack of minerals, is to place these acids within the fatty tissues of the body. Fat acts as a buffer or barrier that keeps the acidic waste as far as possible from the precious organs. Storing acids in the body might be okay for a short while, but when they build up over time and overwhelm the body, they can cause damage to the organs. Not to mention it just sounds gross. I mean, we don't store putrefying trash in our homes; why would we want to store this kind of waste in the body? I'm pretty sure we don't! But it's happening to us on a daily basis because of this unfavorable situation of more acids and less nutrients; the body inevitably becomes overwhelmed and contaminated.

The Body Cannot Burn Acid-Laden Fat

Besides overall calorie consumption, acidic toxic contamination has become one of the main reasons our bodies are obese. Ironically, or maybe not so much, the foods that cause us to be overweight are the very same foods that make our body acidic. We said that our bodies can use fat as another means to buffer the acidic waste trapped within itself. When body fat becomes laden with acids, it becomes impossible to metabolize (burn) without the ability to neutralize the acid waste contained within this body fat first, *before* it can be burned or used for energy. Another possible situation is that the fat is stripped away *before* the contamination is dealt with, which can lead to a devastating amount of contamination being released into the intracellular fluids suddenly, which can have an adverse effect on the organs and structure of the body by causing injury more quickly and severely.

Fortunately, these contaminated foods usually come with a lot of sugars and fats, which can be used to create more body fat in order to provide an ample supply of buffering agent for the continued assault of toxins that these foods carry along with them. However, the result is inevitable: continued weight gain and contamination. Because this buffering technique was never supposed to be a normal function but instead as a temporary, emergency procedure, it again leads to an abundance of body fat (obesity) within the bodies of a lot of us today.

What this means is that if you are overweight and your body is contaminated, it is nearly impossible to lose weight, unless, of course, you start with a detoxification program as part of your weight loss plan, which can be as simple as actually eating the right, healthy, alkalizing foods. This is why some people have success in weight loss: they either consciously or unconsciously eat the correct amount of alkaline foods. At first they are fired up about eating healthy and consume a lot of salad and vegetables, which does exactly what we are talking about, and the weight begins to come off.

Unfortunately, most of the time this does not stick, because the person will often have unbearable cravings for the acidic foods that got them to where they didn't want to be in the first place, instead of continuing to alkalize the body for continued weight loss and health improvement. It is not easy at first, but personally I think that if you follow the all-natural way of life, you will not have to diet in order to stay in shape. Besides, we should not forget that everyone is on a diet; your diet is what you eat every day.

Bad Situation for the Kidneys

The next emergency technique of dealing with a low-mineral store and a low pH (too much acidic waste) is to create ammonia within the kidneys. Ammonia is very alkaline and can be used by the body to neutralize some strong acids. This is, however, a dangerous situation for the kidneys and bladder, as it creates an environment for infection or worse. The kidneys perform upwards of 500 different bodily functions (we think), so it's hard to say just how bad the ramifications of any kidney damage or dysfunction really are going to be.

Having an acidic system is an unhealthy situation for the body. We said an acidic environment leaves us open to dysfunction and disease. When organs are forced to bathe in their own acidic waste or other contaminants, they will be stifled temporarily or will sustain permanent damage. When damage takes place dysfunction is not far behind, when the body's organs aren't functioning properly, we become immune suppressed and left susceptible to more infection and disease.

pH Balance in the Body: Old News

The concept of maintaining the proper pH within the body for essential health originated as far back as the 1930s and earlier. It is believed by me, as well as others, that a low pH or an acidic system is directly or indirectly the cause of all conditions and diseases from acne to Alzheimer's, irritability, psychosis, and arthritis to cancer. It makes sense that this acidic waste causes dysfunction and that dysfunction causes disease and/or injury.

Testing your pH is an easy task that you can do every now and then to help monitor your toxicity level. This is achieved by checking the pH of the urine and saliva. These tests should be conducted in the morning or early in the day and with some added minor calculations, depending on the method you choose—you can measure the pH of your intra-cellular fluid. One tool is to use litmus paper to test the pH of your urine and saliva. A better way might be to purchase some pH testing strips that are for in-vitro use.

Your urine is always acidic, right? Wrong! I have tested in the morning and actually had slightly alkaline readings 7.1–7.2. This happens mostly when I'm in an alkalizing phase of my diet/lifestyle because I'm trying to raise my pH. During normal periods my pH readings for urine in the morning is slightly acidic 6.6–6.8 and can be lower based on nutritional and stress variables.

There are several factors that will affect a pH reading. One thing is not to test at the end of a long workday, as your acid levels will be up from stress and activity. Also you'll want to avoid testing after working out, as this creates a lot of lactic acid. One easy way to test the strength of your mineral stores (pH) is to eat nothing but meat without any vegetables or other alkalizing agents for three days. Then test your urine and saliva in the morning of the fourth day upon waking. If you get a reading of anything higher than 4.5–5, you know that you have low-mineral stores and that the kidneys are making ammonia to neutralize acids, especially if you get a reading of 7 or better. I said previously that I have tested urine above 7, but this was not during a meat-only phase of testing; this was when I was cleansing and was loading up with alkaline minerals, which is what caused the high pH reading.

Another easy way to test your pH is to test your urine upon awakening (first evacuation), along with your saliva. You can add the two together and then divide by two; this will give an average between the two readings. Your average reading between the urine and saliva will be a good indicator of your overall pH; however, if you test three days in a row and average these three average readings by adding them, then dividing by three again, it is usually more accurate, due to some variables in lifestyle and diet. You can also add a second reading on these three days by testing one half hour after breakfast (assuming you eat one) or within two hours of the first test. Continue to add and divide to average these readings in order to find your overall pH level. Theoretically, the more testing you do, the more accurate the results will be.

Alkalize Now and Forever

If you have already successfully cleansed your body and want to maintain your elevated pH level, check it often. If you find that it is low, try to determine what it is about your regime that is causing the reduction in pH (acidity). Next try an alkalizing phase. Alkalizing phase? Yup, that's when you change things for a while, similar to a cleansing, but not necessarily as intense.

Make some minor changes to your diet for a short period of time by excluding meat, any processed foods, and other junk for a few days, all the while adding a lot of extra clean alkaline water and a lot of green alkalizing organic vegetables. (For those of you who don't know, *organic* in this case refers to food, medicine, and cosmetic items that are not made of or do not have any exposure to unnatural chemicals at all throughout their journey from production to our tables and homes, with some variables of course.)

Life will kick your butt. We get stressed out, behind on our deadlines, and we don't always have time to pay attention to a healthy diet or overall health in general. It is during these times that our acidity level goes up. (We will learn how stress and the mind can drastically affect our overall health in upcoming chapters.) This is why it's important to check your pH level on a regular basis. And if you find it low, try to take steps to bring it back up in order to achieve and maintain balance within the body.

Long-term *acidosis* can lead to all sorts of health problems, some of them mild at first and seem to be normal as everyone has these symptoms now and then. If the body becomes heavily acidic over time from prolonged acidic diet and lifestyle, the problems get exponentially worse, as injuries and dysfunction begin to take place. These injuries often go unnoticed, as the symptoms might not so obviously give away their cause.

More Contamination over Time

The longer a body lives, the more it must expose itself to. It must eat, breathe, and drink. The more air we breathe, the more toxins we inhale. The more food we eat, the more contaminants we ingest, same with drinking water. Consuming animal food products that live short lives and are low on the food chain are cleaner choices than ones higher up on the chain that live a long life. Also, animals that have lived a natural, healthy lifestyle are also better food choices, as we are what we eat. Humans are at the top of the food chain and live a long time in comparison to most of the foods we eat. This means that every year, starting at birth, our bodies become more and more contaminated (acidic) due to simply and ironically trying to stay alive and healthy by consuming food and water. You will see this is true as we look at the different stages of acidosis and their symptoms.

Symptom Stages of Acidosis

Mild Symptoms in the Beginning

Food Allergies

Hyperactivity Disorder

Panic Attacks

Pre-menstrual menstrual cramping, anxiety and depression

Poor Sex Drive

Bloating Within the Abdomen

Acne

Agitation

Muscular and Joint Aches and Pains

Poor Circulation Cold Extremities

Dizziness

Fatigue

Indigestion

Irregularity

Hot Urine

Shallow Fast Breathing

Excessive Heartbeat

Heart Murmur

Thrush

Fatigue in the morning

Excess Mucous

Metal Taste

Intermediate Symptoms of Acidosis

Diarrhea

Stuttering

Lack of sensation

Tingling

Sinusitis

Depression

Memory Loss

Confusion

Migraines

Sleeplessness

Herpes

Candida Yeast Infections

RingWorm

Impotence

Cystitis

Urinary Tract Infection

Gastritis

Colitis

Balding

Psoriasis

Problems with Smelling, Tasting, Seeing, Hearing Asthma

Seasonal Allergies

Ear Infections and Aches

Hives

Inflammation

Colds

Flu

Infections

Advanced Symptoms of Acidosis

Arthritis
Osteoporosis
Scleroderma
Leukemia
Tuberculosis
Cancer
Crohn's Disease
Schizophrenia
Learning Deficiencies
Hodgkin's Disease
Lupus
MS
Sarcoidosis

Cancer

All forms of cancer and disease are severe symptoms of lowest pH. If natural or other toxic waste accumulates within the cell, it will turn cancerous and continue to clone itself with this new mutated form of cell. It does this in order to adapt to the acidic environment. This is why cancers can return after being surgically removed. If the acidic environment does not change, cancers will continue to mutate as they did the first time. This is why it is imperative to alkalize your body now with a healthy lifestyle.

John Hopkins University has discovered a link between a lack of oxygen and a cell turning cancerous (John Hopkins, 2011). They discovered that a cell with less oxygen adapts by turning cancerous and uses more sugar for energy than oxygen. It has long been known that cancer feeds on sugars to stay alive. When the cell becomes contaminated, waste products will block the cell receptors, preventing proper oxygen and informational flow. Just as we have already learned, the higher the pH in your water, the more oxygen it contains, which gives us three benefits: alkalization, oxygenation, and with the added benefits of ions, anti aging, and conductive properties.

Obesity

We talked about the three different emergency procedures our bodies perform in order to deal with accumulating acids. Here we are concerned with the body using fat as a buffer. If your body's first defense (due to either the availability of fat, body chemistry, or genetics) is to buffer these acids with fat, then over time your body will continue to accumulate fat, as it is a necessary tool in maintaining a safe distance between the organs and the acidic waste.

It becomes impossible to metabolize this fat, as it is laden with acidic contaminants. To try to burn this fat is a problem for two reasons: one is that it is too toxic to be used. Next is that because of the buildup of toxins, there is insufficient alkali and oxygen, both of which are required to achieve this breaking down of the fatty tissues (metabolizing). This is why cleansing your body and alkalizing the correct way will cause the "side effect" of losing weight.

Diabetes

Diabetes's scientific term is called *diabetic keto-acidosis*. I think the name says it all here. This is one of the many injuries that can take place due to acid waste buildup somewhere in the body. In this case, we are referring to the pancreas. It is not as simple as the pancreas being exposed to toxins in general that causes diabetes. Because the overall pH of the digestive system is monitored and manipulated by the pancreas as it is the gateway to the digestive system, it makes sense that in this world of highly acidic waste that the pancreas would be one of the most susceptible organs to dysfunction behind the liver. As usual genetics will decide which dysfunction will take place in different individuals, due to toxic contamination. Obviously some of us won't get diabetes, but we could get something else instead.

Hypertension

Hypertension is very common today among adults and even young people. This can manifest itself three ways: first, capillaries become restricted by surrounding inflammation (physical stresses). Second, blood vessels become clogged with acidic waste, decreasing diameter, increasing blood pressure. Finally, the decreased blood flow and acidic environment cause an insufficient oxygen supply to the cellular tissues of the body, which needless to say is thought to be one of the basic dysfunctions causing all disease today.

Hypotension

Hypotension is the weakening of the heart muscles due to a waste buildup within the cells of the heart muscle tissues. The lack of nutrients and ions as usual is the overall culprit. This ailment as well as gout are great examples of how simply drinking structured, alkaline, ionic water can help alleviate these conditions.

Kidney Ailments and Kidney Stones

Calcium deposits go hand in hand with acidity. When the body's environment is acidic, there is an increase in wastes to deal with. The kidneys' job is to deal with eliminating these wastes, but if there are a lot of acids consistently, this will put a strain on them and can cause all kinds of kidney ailments.

Kidney stones are usually made of calcium that solidifies in the body after being used for neutralization. Typically they occur within or are filtered out by the kidneys. When the body is acidic, it is often dehydrated as well. After robbing calcium from the bones, this heavily saturated solution (urine) due to the lack of water and buildup of wastes can solidify and leave behind stones.

Gout

Gout happens when calcium accumulates in the capillary blood vessels of the hands and feet due to a buildup of uric acid. This is another example of calcium that was robbed from the bones for neutralization purposes, later being deposited somewhere in the body. Normally, gout occurs in toe, knee, and finger joints. Consuming alkaline water is one of the best treatments for alleviating this ailment.

Chronic Constipation

Because of poor diet and the resulting acidity and waste buildup, combined with a lack of hydration, the intestines become compacted and sluggish. This is due to the lack of hydrating foods and water, which adds dysfunction to the digestive system. To remedy this, drink lots and lots of healthy water, as this is the best choice to get things started as well as making better food choices in the future.

The more research you do on the subject, you will find this to be true. All disease and dysfunction starts with the body's inability to clean itself due to lack of nutrients, which leads to waste buildup and low pH. This condition later leads to the breakdown of the body's tissues and organs. As this is true, we must draw the conclusion that taking steps now to correct this unbalance in the body is the key to success in getting and staying healthy.

Contamination from Water and Air

What types of contaminants are getting into the body? Where do they come from? How do we avoid them? And more importantly, how do we get rid of them?

Accidental and Intentional Contaminations

Well water gone unchecked can contain all kinds of pollutants like radon gas, arsenic, lead, and other heavy metals, as well as MTBE contaminants from petroleum products like gasoline. These could be considered accidental contaminations. Sometimes, however, there are contaminants placed in the drinking water on purpose.

Water and water-based beverages can be contaminated with pollutants unknowingly, or they can be put there intentionally. For example, we have all heard of a boil-water order in a town or city due to a biological contamination in the drinking water; this would denote an accidental contamination. But municipal water almost always has chlorine and sometimes contains fluoride and other intentionally placed chemical substances within it. Water quality varies from region to region in municipal and private water sources. Our country's infrastructure has become dilapidated over the years, especially the water systems, with a grade (rating) of D-, which does not help with the ongoing water quality problem (ASCE, 2012).

Effects of Chlorine in Municipal Water Sources

You hear all the time that to drink a lot of water is good for the body. Well it is! *Except* when the water is contaminated! Drinking too much of it, or any of it, can be detrimental to your health, to say the least. Contaminated water is almost always acidic (there are alkaline contaminants as well) and therefore contributes to an acidic environment in the body.

Chlorine is used in the water supply in order to keep it safe. Although necessary to keep bacteria and other pathogens from contaminating the water supply and further infect the people drinking it, it still should be considered unfavorable to consume or clean your body with.

Is Fluoride Good or Bad?

Fluoride is another item that is intentionally placed in the drinking water. It has been debated for years that using fluoride will help prevent tooth decay, but it is also known by the medical community that too much fluoride is bad for your bones and teeth (fluorosis). The debate has always been whether or not the risks to our overall heath outweigh the benefits of tooth decay prevention. Any risk to my health at all to me is unacceptable, as there are safer ways to maintain good oral health.

There have been studies done between countries that use fluoride versus countries that do not. There was found to be no difference in the decline of tooth decay over the last fifty-plus years between the countries that use fluoride verses the ones that don't. The same held true that tooth decay had been reduced with *and* without the use of fluoride, at an even rate (Dr. Bill Osmunson DDS, 2012).

Fluoride is or was considered a drug, which means they deliberately put drugs in the drinking water! Sounds crazy, but it's true. As far as I know, especially considering I am a plumbing contractor, there are no drug fact labels listed on the faucet in your kitchen, so how do you know how much to drink? And did the local government regulating these water characteristics expect you to drink another source of water once you have reached your maximum daily dose of fluoride somehow. Or are we to drink as much as we want regardless of the fluoride content?

On the back of your fluoride toothpaste, the directions tell you to use a pea-sized amount of paste, as a dosage of the drug sodium fluoride, when brushing your teeth (in the commercial they show a huge portion covering the entire brush head). This equals the typical dose of fluoride contained within an eight-ounce glass of tap water, which has been treated with fluoride. Further along in the drug facts warning label on the toothpaste is the statements, "Do not swallow. If you do, contact a poison control center." How does that make sense? The same .25 mg of sodium fluoride in your eight-ounce glass of *drinking water* should *not be swallowed* when it's in your toothpaste. Plus, I'm pretty sure we were told to drink more than one glass of water a day. I am a firm believer that if you can't eat it, don't put it on your skin. The concept of being okay in your mouth but not if you swallow is even more ridiculous than the idea that it is okay on your skin, but not in your mouth (Dr. Bill Osmunson DDS, 2012).

What's worse is the fluoride-treated nursery water meant to be used for making baby formula. Using distilled water for making baby formula is a good idea. Some people think it's strange, as they have only heard of using this type of water in appliances; however, when you mix distilled water with formula, it is no longer distilled. Distilled water is boiled off then the steam vapors are collected so they will condensate and then can be collected as a liquid, which is now free from any contamination that was in the original water; this part is good. But the addition of fluoride to the water that is to be used for mixing baby formula doesn't make sense to me. I was under the impression that the formula companies already put together the most advanced recipe for the infant, which leads to the question: Why would we need to add anything but water? All these questions reinforce that breastfeeding is the safest and best way (the all-natural way) to feed your baby.

Although the most obvious sources of fluoride are toothpaste and fluoridated water, more people are actually exposed to these toxic forms of fluoride through the consumption of non-organic foods, due to the fluoride-based pesticides being used today within this type of food production. Despite the controversy surrounding the use of fluoride within the water supply, still there are more than 60 percent of these water supplies being treated today with fluoride. There is a good chance you might be consuming fluoridated water on a daily basis (Tuberose, 2012).

Fluoride is also one of the main ingredients of Prozac and Sarin (nerve gas), as well as pesticides, herbicides, anesthetics, hypnotics, psychiatric drugs, and other military nerve gases (Tuberose, 2012).

It is believed by myself and many others that the addition of fluoride into the water supply system was originally thought of by some corporate officials from the manufacturing sector. The fluoride was used in the manufacturing of aluminum and many other products, which caused there to be a lot of fluoride *waste* to get rid of. They were able to convince lawmakers that adding it to the drinking water supply was a great idea for helping to keep the populace healthy with strong teeth., which really was a cover up of more covert experiments of subjugating a populace with the use of fluoride (Tuberose, 2012).

What Water Source Is Safe to Drink?

Well, how do I know if the water I'm drinking is healthy or even safe? There are water filters to filter out the bad stuff. So

I could consume filtered water. Problem is, filtered water is not a good solution, unless you buy a really expensive filter. If the filter doesn't work well, it will leave contaminants and pathogenic microbes behind. If the filter works too well, it will remove too much of the necessary minerals that should be left in the water; either way, it leaves the water in an unhealthy state.

Any canned or bottled drink other than water is going to be filtered. Corporations aren't going to chance an inconsistency in their product by not using purified water as a base for their drink product, as this could affect taste and ultimately sales. Okay that's good, right? At least it's clean. The next problem typically is that after filtering out any possible existing contaminants, they add other contaminants of their own such as HFCS (high fructose corn syrup), preservatives, artificial colors, artificial sugars, modified sugars, artificial flavors and sweeteners, phosphates, and other acidifying agents.

There are some healthy choices out there, but these aren't as readily available in most grocery stores, let alone convenient stores. This means your average soda, fruit, or energy drink you find readily available today contains most, if not all of the previously stated toxic ingredients. Even organic fruit juice, due to the sugar content and the "dead" fruit, is not good to consume as a form of hydration or nutrition. It should be limited to adding flavor to your water on occasion or as a vitamin C source. Organic colas, fruit-flavored sodas, spritzers, teas, and other water-based fruit juice drinks are available at your local health food store but again should be limited in consumption, due to high sugar content, and should not be considered a healthy form of hydration. Some of our older folks might remember going to the soda jerk to get a soda, and it was considered a sweet treat or a dessert, like getting an ice cream today—not a healthy form of hydration.

Distilled Water Is Clean Water

Distilled water is not a good choice for regular hydration, despite the purity. Distilled or purified water is okay to drink (if you can stand it) for a short period of time, such as a day or two. The reason for doing this would be for cleansing purposes only, not as a means of hydrating your body on a regular basis. Just like making baby formulas, it is not only safe but a good idea to use distilled water to make other types of beverages like coffee, tea, cocoa, pasta, rice, smoothies, or any other food that you add water to or cook with.

Is Purified Water Safe to Drink?

Drinking distilled, reverse osmosis, or purified water is dangerous on a long-term basis, as it is caustic to the body. Because it is devoid of minerals due to the decontamination process, this water would have to be digested by the body before it can be absorbed. Another downfall of this characteristic is that this water is almost always acidic and as a result contains more CO_2 than O_2. As we know, CO_2 is a waste product that the body tries to eliminate consistently through the lungs by exhaling (acidic waste).

Digesting Water?

We mentioned digesting water; the first part of this digestion would be to warm the water to the temperature of the body so it can be absorbed, which is why it is better to drink water used for hydrating purposes at room temperature or warmed. Next is to structure the water in order to create small enough groups of water molecules, which enable them to pass through the cellular walls (colloidal). Non-colloidal water cannot be used by the body and must be structured first. This is where the problem arises through the body's process for structuring the water.

What this means to us is if we consume this type of purified water on a regular basis, it can further strain our already low or depleted mineral stores. Purified water can actually dissolve bones and joints due to the acidic qualities. Things like osteoporosis and arthritis can occur due to the stripping or dissolving actions of the ultra-filtered water. It is very important to drink structured, mineral-laden, alkaline ionic water. Drinking alkaline water helps maintain a higher pH level in the body because we are adding more alkaline elements, rather than acidic ones, to our body's intracellular fluids (environment) by doing so.

Identifying Healthy Water Sources

Sounds good, but how do I achieve this? How do I know if the water I am drinking is healthy? There are some water-bottling companies out there who can provide you with a decent drink of water by filtering the water several times and later adding trace elements (minerals) to enhance the taste. Their efforts will usually bring you a drink of water that is clean and neutral, but this water still does not offer all of the beneficial characteristics healthy water should possess. This is the absolute minimum standard of water that I will consume; however, I only drink this kind of water when I run out of my own water. While I am away from home, I carry two forty-two-ounce stainless steel containers of my special water with me at all times, which at 220 pounds of body weight is a good amount for the workday. I drink more in the morning and at night as well.

There are other healthier choices out there; some options are waters that contain extra alkaline elements in order to raise the pH beyond neutral to ranges from 7.5 to 9. This is advantageous, as it helps facilitate a higher pH within the body when consumed on a regular basis. Water that is alkaline contains more oxygen. The higher the pH of the water, the more oxygen the water contains as they are directly related. This is a better choice, but these waters still lack one more important characteristic.

Benefits of Ions or Electrolytes

There is one last property of healthy water that we should consider. We want to know if the water is ionic. What this very simply means is that the elements that are structuring and alkalizing the water are negatively charged with an extra electron. This is beneficial as this property of the water helps conduct electricity. Yes, electricity. Your body is electric; it has a frequency, which is a direct representation of electrical activity. Einstein and Edison proved this in the early 1900s (Kevin Trudeau, 2009).

Ionic water helps facilitate better communication between the body's systems by readily giving up electrons that neutralize free radicals and promote electrical flow. A free radical is a particle or ion that is positively charged. Positively charged ions want to be neutralized, in other words not positive or negative. Because free radicals, or positively charged ions, want to be neutralized, they steal the first electron they can find. This is disadvantageous to the body, as the robbing of electrons actually means the robbing of energy and information that is trying to be transmitted between the brain and the many different types of neurons within the body.

When a free radical meets up with a negative ion (electrolyte), the negative ion gives up its extra electron, which leaves the two particles neutral, therefore preventing the disturbance of electrical flow within the body. When the body's electrical systems are undisturbed, the body can and will function more efficiently, further allowing the rest of your body's systems to function more efficiently. This is why drinks that contain electrolytes boast the ability to give you more energy and quicker recovery time after exercising or playing hard.

Achieving Healthy Water Sources

This all sounds so overwhelming, but it's true! The reality is that there are very few beverages out there—in my opinion—that are safe to drink. Even bottled water is dangerous due to the unknown. So how does the average person achieve safe and healthy forms of hydration?

There are a few ways to do this; one is to purchase what's called an oxygen cooler. This is really a fancy name for a water filter that has the ability to remove all the contaminants and as many of the acidic elements as desired, creating a clean, alkaline, ionic drinking water with a variable pH level of 7.5–10, depending on the setting. These filters also create an acidic wastewater that can be used as a cleanser in your home. These filters are state of the art, as they have the ability to charge the elements as well, giving you the ionic properties desired. The one drawback in the case is that they are very expensive but are still worth the investment if you can afford it (Enagic, 2012).

Creating Healthy Water Sources

Another means of achieving pure, alkaline, ionic water that is easy and affordable, is to "engineer" it yourself. To achieve this, first we start with distilled water, which can be purchased from your local drug store or your local water-delivery service (not all water services offer distilled delivered, but some do and they are out there). Then we add our own trace and alkaline elements to structure and alkalize the water.

These water-based mineral supplements can be purchased from your local health food store or online. Be sure that it is a two-part mix—one for structure and one for alkalizing. This is the method I chose because I like the idea of starting with distilled water, which we know is totally devoid of anything other than H2O (ultra-purified). The mineral supplements that I buy are reasonably priced and negatively charged. So in the end, my family ends up with perfectly-engineered water for around one-dollar a gallon United States and less when I hit the sales right. Another benefit is that after you structure the water, you can adjust the pH by adding more or less of the second alkalizing part of the mix. As you raise your pH, you may not need to drink water as high in pH as you did in the beginning, because when your pH levels are higher, it takes less alkali to neutralize these weaker acids.

ORP: What Does It Mean?

ORP, or oxygen reduction potential, refers to the ability of ionic alkaline water to act as an antioxidant. The reason that ionic alkaline water contains more oxygen is because of the chemical transformation that takes place within the water molecule when we change it from acidic to alkaline. We all know that water is represented by the chemical symbol H2O. This tells us that there are two hydrogen atoms to every oxygen atom, giving us a 2-to-1 ratio. When water is structured and alkalized with ionic alkaline elements, the water changes to the chemical state represented by the symbol OH- (Ian Blair Hamilton, 2012).

This does two things; first it doubles the amount of oxygen in the water, which along with the help of the hydrogen atom burns calories more efficiently, giving us more energy. Second this gives us the antioxidant capabilities of the OH- molecule, as it is ready to give up the extra electron used to neutralize free radicals within the body, which would otherwise use the oxygen molecule to oxidize or age the body's tissues.

An ion is a particle with either a positive or negative charge within its chemical makeup. Free radicals are positively charged particles (ions) that lack an electron. An electrolyte is a negatively charged particle (ions) with an extra electron; it is this extra electron that is given up to the free radical leaving the two particles now neutral, or not positive or negative and no longer an ion. Free radicals mixed with oxygen will cause oxidation or rusting of the organs, causing premature aging (Ian Blair Hamilton, 2012).

Always remember that we are made mostly of water and that the body uses water for *all* of its functions. Next to our own blood, water is the next most important component of life. Please consider the water you drink imperative for staying healthy.

Cellular Waste from Normal Functions

Under normal circumstances, the body creates waste from the metabolizing of food. When the mitochondria within the cell burn glucose for energy, naturally there are waste products produced. We eat and poop on a cellular level as well as a human one. These waste products can wreak havoc on the body if left behind to build up; however, there are far worse contaminants these days within the body.

At the same time, ironically, the nutritional value within the food that we eat today has diminished to a level not ample for keeping up with the normal body wastes, never mind the overwhelming amount of toxins our bodies are exposed to today, so much so that most of us are suffering from malnutrition (unless of course, you consume higher quality foods in the correct amounts on a regular basis). The problem with this is that the body uses nutrients (and water) to cleanse itself, but due to the low nutrition within our food today, our resulting mineral stores are low, and our bodies are unable to perform their cleansing techniques. So we are left with a double-edged sword—more contamination combined with less nutrition gives us a low pH (acidic bodily environment), which leaves an environment fit for disease.

Environmental Sources of Contamination

What types of contaminants are getting into the body, and where do they come from? First there are environmental contaminants such as air pollution. Air pollution can account for up to 2 million premature deaths per year, according to the World Health Organization. They have discovered this by gathering information from over 1,100 cities over 91 countries (Wendy Koch, 2011).

It contains pollution particulates that vary in volume (PPM) depending on the day and geographical location. It can contain many types of carcinogens and other compounds that are unfavorable and toxic to the body and lungs.

Sources of Air Pollution

These can come from factories manufacturing chemicals, vehicles spewing fumes from burning fossil fuels, or, worse yet, chemically enhanced fossil fuels like rocket fuel. Also the air in your house can be filled with contaminants and free radicals from cleansers, appliances, and building products like formaldehyde-laden fiberglass insulation, not to mention lead paint and asbestos and others that we can't even conceive of, as well.

Air fresheners contain manmade chemicals and can also place dangerous chemicals into the air. A better choice is always a natural one, using *pure*, therapeutic essential oils for freshening *and* decontaminating the air in your home. We tend not to think about air pollution problems and causes unless it is bad enough to see. Air pollution is rarely seen, felt, or smelled. It is a typically a silent, invisible health risk, gone unnoticed and unchecked by most people.

Contamination from Food

How Foods Contaminate the Body

Consuming food is one of the most obvious ways our bodies becomes contaminated and should be subject to scrutiny by us. The food industry would sell you a bag of smashed lips and toes to eat if they knew you'd buy it. And they do! Believe me! It's unfathomable to me some of the things that people eat, or that I've eaten in the past for that matter. Keep in mind it's a hundred times worse for your pet unless you do something to correct that, as well.

Our dog eats organic dog food and drinks healthy water; as a result, he has had a clean bill of health every year at the vet since he started—"Hobbes." The cheapest pet foods are made of some of the most dangerous ingredients.

There are many different stages to consider for the production of our food, from being grown to when it makes it to your table. The initial stage is when the food is grown; the next phase is when the food is harvested; from there the food is transported and stored, oftentimes only to be transported again to factories. This is where the food is processed, only to be packaged and stored again, later transported to the supermarket where it will be stored again for another period of time, and finally you will transport it from the market to your house, and store it again before finally consuming it at the dinner table. The average meal in America today comes from 1,400 miles away (Robert Kenner, 2008).

Most of us understand that fast and junk foods are bad for you with the obvious reasons being high fat, sugar, calories, and the processing involved. These facts don't surprise most people; however, there are many other reasons that these and other types of foods that are being sold today, even carrying the label healthy, are dangerous to consume.

How Greed Affects Food Quality

With agribusiness and greed in big business, food has transformed from a green, wholesome, vibrant, life-giving wealth of sustenance to a for-profit, brown, dead, life-taking plague! Food is often produced with nothing more in mind other than maximizing profit no matter what the cost to people's health and financial welfare, as well as polluting, straining, and stripping the environment of its divine gifts. We will soon learn that these practices are not sustainable for people or the planet.

So Many Food Additives to Choose From

There are literally thousands of additives and preservatives available to food producers, which are used in food production and storage. These products are created and used to keep the foods from breaking down as well as inhibit the growth of bacteria, mold, and yeast. Some of the commonly used food additives and preservatives are amino acid compounds, ammonium carbonates, aluminum silicate, sodium nitrate, butylated hydrozyttoluene (BHT), butylated hydroxyanisole (BHA), monosodium glutamate (MSG), sugars (typically modified), potassium bromate and sorbate, sodium benzoate, etc.

Artificial colors are also added to foods, despite the dangers, only to create an appealing look. Here are some examples of these substances: erythrosine (red), cantaxanthin (orange), amaranth (Azoic red), tartrazine (Azoic yellow), and annatto bixine (yellow-orange). All of these chemicals are either known (toxins) carcinogens or are suspected to be (Sustainable Table, 2012).

Modified and Trans Fats

Trans fats and modified fats—are they any different? The answer is no. We've all heard of hydrogenated fats or trans fats, and we have all heard by now of the health ramifications that these trans fats have caused (some towns and states have actually outlawed the use of these trans fats). These trans fats are in reality "modified" fats, but they are modified in this case with the use of the hydrogen molecule (hydrogenated oils).

All the bad press and the evil reputation that the term *hydrogenated fats* or *trans fats* have earned led to an awareness and further avoidance of the food choices that contain these fats. This potentially hurt sales in two ways. First, the company was selling fewer products because people didn't want to buy or consume them due to these dangerous fats contained within them. Second, they had to change their ingredients, which causes a temporary increase in logistics and further an overall increase in cost due to the use of the new replacement ingredients.

To remedy this, the food manufacturers (chemists in the food industry) have already and will continue to simply come up with new ways to modify fats and other foods once again, which will be given a new name by the industry that we will be unfamiliar with. This will make it harder for us to facilitate the ability to avoid these new, potentially hazardous foods. As always, the best choice is organic. Due to the unknown and unavoidable, even certified organic foods can still contain some unnatural substances. These substances are either a necessity for environmental issues such as the introduction of foreign insects from another country's fruit or substances that are introduced unavoidably through accidental exposure. The reason these unnatural, unhealthy techniques (non-organic) are used by manufacturers is, of course, to make more money. Apparently doing things the healthy way costs more to achieve. And as always, there will be a certain amount of deceit within the organic world of food products, as dishonorable people will manipulate the system to suit their needs one way or another; however, they have less room to do it in with the regulations in organics.

So the point here, once again, is that the truth holds true; any chemical substance created or altered by man through the modification of existing chemical substances or elements can be and is most likely harmful for human exposure, because these substances were not part of a healthy lifestyle during evolution. Because of this, our bodies have not yet learned how to deal with or how to use them. This combined with a lack of nutrition and hydration leads us to the overwhelming health problems of today.

Problems with Meats

Cows, pigs, and chickens are raised at an accelerated rate initially by means of hormones, antibiotics, other pharmaceuticals, and more recently through genetic manipulation (GMOs). They are placed within environments full of disease and stress, completely devoid of familiar, natural surroundings, creating a new, potentially unhealthy form of animal and resulting meat product. These animals are not immune to the exposure to unhealthy foods either. They are often fed the same unnatural, chemically toxic, modified foods that we are exposed to on a daily basis only worse because they have no choice in the matter. They eat what we give them.

Cows are jammed onto feedlots where they are fed corn, sugars, meat fillers (not eaten by cows naturally), and other unnatural foods. These things were not meant to be part of their diets. Crowding leaves them unable to eat grass in a pasture, which is what they've done for thousands, even millions of years. Most living creatures of the world do not like to live crammed together in small spaces. As a community develops, oftentimes you will see animals having to relocate to other areas because we have encroached on their territory. A lion and his pride need a lot of area to hunt and live on in order to survive. Some animals are social, and they like to live among themselves, but they still want room to move around and be free from other species' habitats. It is part of their natural lifestyle. The same is true for the animals that we are going to eat; they too want to spread out with room to walk around and have the ability to eat and poop in two separate places.

These feedlots are harboring lake-size plumes of urine and fecal matter that leech out into the adjacent ground waters and farmlands, contributing to groundwater contamination and secondary bacterial contamination of produce. The unnatural diets lead to higher bacteria counts within the cows' digestive systems as well, this being caused by the lack of grass consumption (green vegetables) and the addition of chemicals and sugar to the diet, which lead to infection and disease in the animals, as well as contaminating the resulting meat with E. coli.

Besides poor diet and stress for the animals that causes illness, some farmers implemented rBST hormones in order to get more milk out of each cow. This was naturally procured and instigated by the pharmaceutical company that created the hormone. It doesn't take long before the hormones cause even more infections and tumors within the food population. The cows' udders are being pumped longer and more rapidly, as this is the promised result. They become infected, adding bacteria, puss, and infection to the milk supply (rBST has been linked to accelerating the growth of breast and other cancers) (Robert Cohen, 1997).

In order to battle the onslaught of microbes causing health problems for the cows, the use of antibiotics was implemented. Over time and with continued use in millions of cows, this resulted in the evolution of more anti-bacterial resistant bacterial strains. These microbes that were causing disease within the cows were forced to mutate into stronger versions of themselves in order to survive the battle. This is what gave us new, more deadly forms of E. coli and other microbes. These new deadly forms are consistently getting into our food and water sources and have become resistant to antibiotics due to overuse, not only in cows but in humans as well.

Bacteria Found in Meat

There were at one time up to and more than 100 slaughterhouses in the country butchering cows in order to meet the demand for beef. Today there are fewer than five (this doesn't count the small independent growers and butchers, grass fed, organic, etc.) slaughtering most of the beef cows that we consume at an alarming rate. These kill lines are run too quickly, oftentimes by inept personnel; all the while there exists elevated bacteria levels within the intestines and fecal matter of the cows. This makes the possibility of contamination of the resulting beef more likely. Massive recalls and possible deaths are more common today than ever from tainted meat (Robert Kenner, 2008).

What Kind of Chicken Are *You* Eating?

Recently the use of hormones has been outlawed in some areas of the food production industry. Again we saw the health ramifications to the animals along with the resulting consequences, later leading to bad press for the food producers and finally loss of profit. But these changes aren't made for the good, nor are they implemented before the remedy has been achieved. Since we cannot use hormones any longer to produce more meat, we now instead use the technique of genetic modification.

Not only did the food manufacturers come up with a solution for more meat without hormones, but it had another benefit as well: if you use hormones for production, you must continue to purchase these hormones and treat each and every animal that you raise. This carries with it a substantial overhead cost than if you genetically modify an animal. Theoretically you only have to change the first one and let nature do the rest from there, unless of course nature won't allow your modification to facilitate the continued procreation of this new modified creature. (A mule is the successful mating between a horse and a donkey. However, their offspring typically cannot reproduce).

Chickens raised for meat production have been genetically modified and grow so quickly that after only six weeks of growth, they can no longer walk. They are crammed into cages so small they can barely raise a wing or move around at all without trampling each other, which they do. Their beaks are cut or burnt off in order to prevent the birds from pecking each other, thus taking away their ability to eat normally or defend themselves as they would have normally been able to do.

Cage-free birds do not necessarily get to walk around in an open pasture and eat grass; it simply means, through the official definition from the government, that each bird has two-square feet of area within the facility per bird. Because more room to roam means more land, which creates more overhead, these fowl are unable to frolic and eat grass that is probably the best medicine for them. If your body is dysfunctional in any way due to contamination from poor diet, it will cause one kind of physical stress, which inhibits the ability to manage mental stresses and therefore can cause you to become stressed in every way! (Molly Watson, 2012).

When stress levels are high, be it physical, mental or both, the immune system becomes suppressed. When the immune system is suppressed, stress levels are high and infection levels are increased. Stress and illness go hand in hand—true for us, true for animals. Mental stress causes acidosis, acidosis causes physical stress, and physical stress can lead to mental stress; it is a vicious cycle. As always, we ignore immune suppression and have fought infection with the use of antibiotics within chickens as well. The resulting food products end up being the opposite of what they should be: unhealthy instead of good for you.

Eating Fish Is Good, Right?

Farm-raised fish have become more popular today in the fish-producing and marketing sectors. This type of fish production was created through the necessity to remedy overfishing. However, there are certain techniques used to farm fish that can be close to the lifestyle and development of natural fish, but there are other techniques implemented that do not resemble a natural life for these fish. Typically doing the right thing costs more money, and when there is a way to do it cheaper, most if not all of the time these more cost-effective techniques are implemented to increase the bottom line. With farm-raised fish, like the production of cows, the issue is how much area they will use to produce a certain number of living product.

Genetic manipulation, if not already common practice in the fish industry, will be soon. There is not as much information available to us divulging the use of such techniques by food producers as of yet. The FDA does *not* require food companies to divulge to the consumer whether the food products that they are selling have genetically modified ingredients or not. Hopefully soon they will, but as of right now, the only way to be *almost* positive is to buy only certified organic or wild-caught food choices.

As always, due to economics (greed), there is the need to produce as much food as possible in the smallest area of land, resulting in the lowest cost. As a result, fish are fed a poor, unnatural diet and are crammed together, swimming in polluted waters. Some of these species might have migration instincts but will not have the ability to swim long distances and to different regions. Their captivity prevents the fish from living an all-natural lifestyle in many other ways.

Less Living, Less Contamination

But eating fish is good for you, right? What about omega-3s? Small, oily, wild-caught fish are an essential part of a well-balanced diet. These fish contain quality proteins combined with fatty acids, both of which are good for overall health. Sardines and herring are but a few of these small, oily fish. Because they are low on the food chain and do not live as long as bigger fish, they do not have the chance to become as contaminated as do other fish species that are higher on the food chain.

Deep ocean fish like haddock, swordfish, tuna, and other lager fish, due to pollution, have become toxic with heavy metals. These fish can still be consumed but should be limited to six ounces a week for healthy adults (twelve and up). Children are more susceptible to the effects of heavy metals, as well as people who are ill and the elderly. In these cases you may want to refrain from these fish choices altogether, especially if you already have some kind of neurological disorder such as Parkinson's, Alzheimer's, ADD, ADHD, autism, etc.

Is Shellfish Safe to Consume?

Fish fit for consumption must have scales and fins. I believe the reason is because they are otherwise unhealthy, due to contamination, regardless of pollution. After all, they are bottom feeders, and we all know what ends up at the bottom—the more dominant species' excrement. I enjoy some shellfish once or twice a year, but I also realize that it is junk food when I do. You'll want to make sure if you choose to eat any of this type of fish that it is cooked thoroughly, due to the possibility of microbial (parasitic) contamination, as well as realize the existence of other types of contamination old and new.

Pork and Pork Products: Good or Bad?

Since pigs are creatures that consume feces, this leads to extensive contamination, especially parasitic, as the average lifecycle of a parasite usually includes a ride from the bowels of one creature to the belly of another. So it seems like pork products are the perfect place to encounter many different types of parasites. After being consumed by the pigs through feces, these parasites can be passed on to humans, who consume these swine products, through their infected tissues. Always cook pork well in order to kill off any parasitic contaminations (160 degrees F).

Another reason pork products are less favorable is that pork has a high-fat content. As we know, animal fat is laden with acidic contaminants. High-fat diets, especially animal fats, are well known to be unhealthy. This is another reason why beef and pork are considered more dangerous than chicken and fish and should be limited and of high quality; organic and wild caught being the best.

Unhealthy Environment, Unhealthy Animals

Animals raised within crammed spaces have high stress and disease and typically do not get the nutrition that they need; therefore, they themselves are unhealthy. Consuming unhappy, unhealthy animals is, in fact, making us unhealthy and, yes, unhappy. It only makes sense that if you eat unhealthy food you will be unhealthy.

And now you know the other reason why we should treat animals with care and respect, even if we are going to eat them! Our food needs to be given proper care and environment, as do we, in order to be and remain healthy. Why not treat these animals like kings while they are alive, as they are going to give their lives to us in the end? So even if you are not an animal lover, you're still going want to make sure the person growing your food *is* and that they have respect for the environment as well (cruelty free).

Kobe Beef is a beef product made from a bovine species in Asia. These animals are massaged and given one beer a day to reduce stress. They are fed an all natural diet and are very happy and healthy. This beef costs upwards of five hundred dollars a pound and is used to make beef pâté and other high-end beef dishes (Meat Man, 2012).

Produce Is Always Good for You, Right?

What could possibly be wrong with fresh produce? Anything with DNA can be genetically manipulated by man, even produce. Now when I say genetically modified, I don't mean cross-pollinating different types of fruits and vegetables (although I prefer heirlooms), as this is okay. When you cross-pollinate different vegetation, you are asking God if this works or not, is this okay? God will then respond with the correct answer, and you can be sure that it will be something your body will recognize as food.

When we genetically alter the DNA of food, we are telling God that we know better than He does, which is foolish arrogance. We have no idea, as this is basically a new tool in science and the industry of food, what the health ramifications will be from consuming these GMOs at all, never mind on a regular basis. Personally these are especially scary techniques, and I do not want to be exposed to them at all.

GMOs, Pesticides, Herbicides, and Others

Besides GMOs, you have to worry about pesticides and herbicides, which have shown to cause a plethora of health problems, more than we realize I'm sure. Always remember that the herbicides or pesticides are not included in the ingredient labels on your food, even though they are included in the production of the food item. So any processed food that contains a particular food type as a base (such as grains in cereal) that has been exposed to herbicides and or pesticides, which possibly still contain residue from said chemicals, the food producers do not have to tell you that they are there when describing the ingredients of the resulting food product, nor do they have to tell you if it's a GMO (Deyanda Flint, 2012).

Frequent bacterial infestations of the world's produce are mostly caused directly or indirectly by animal feces, which have become a problem within the world of ground water as well. However, if you can't give plants antibiotics, how do you deal with these microbes? You can always wash them in chlorinated water (tap water), which can turn some vegetables into poison. Or you can throw them in the microwave (irradiation), which renders the life force of the plant kaput.

Unfortunately, these are the things that are done on a regular basis to our food, and make no mistake, it's why we are sick. It's also a major contributor to the fact that the environment is polluted. These corporate practices include the centralizing of production, which not only takes business away from small to large family owned and operated farms but also has strained and polluted the environment. As a result, these conditions have made it more difficult to purchase responsibly grown, healthy food.

Other Sources of Contamination

Is Cleaning Your Home Killing You?

Household cleansers, laundry detergent, and dish detergents can contain dangerous chemicals that we expose ourselves to every day. This is not thought about by many people, yet could be a dangerous source of contamination to our bodies. The idea of toxic dish detergent being dangerous seems reasonable since we put food on the pans and dishes that contain residue from chemical cleansers, but what about household cleaners?

There are a few examples of cleaning surfaces that we do not come into contact with, such as the toilet. It seems there is no danger to use strong chemicals on the bowl, but what about the seat? More importantly, what about the environment? Most of us flush our toilets into our backyard. If the effluent waters are laden with chemicals, this can, needless to say, be unhealthy to your septic system and the environment.

Countertops, tables, and other surfaces that we and our food come into contact with need to be free of toxic cleaners before we touch them or they touch our food. Some of the so-called "convenient" cleaning wipes, when used to clean household surfaces, need to be rinsed away after use in order to make the surfaces safe for exposure, especially by the immune-deficient, elderly, and young children. Naturally they have placed this fact in tiny, illegible writing at the bottom of the screen during the commercial, hoping you won't notice, as this information makes the idea of convenience ridiculous.

Steam is an effective way to kill bacteria on surfaces within your home without the use of expensive, dangerous chemicals. Also, there are special blends of essential oils for cleansing; which is another all-natural way to disinfect yourself, your home, and goods. Even the popular brand name companies are starting to create more plant-based cleansers to choose from.

How Can Laundry Detergent Be Dangerous?

Maybe you know someone who cannot use a particular detergent on their clothes because it causes skin irritation or they have an allergic reaction. Or maybe you were worried about the sensitive skin of your newborn baby and decided to use a "free and clear" version of a brand-name detergent. So it's seems we are concerned of the effects detergent has on our skin, but we need to understand that contamination of the skin doesn't stop there, at the skin, as the skin is a permeable barrier of the internal body.

Our skin is not a safe, impermeable barrier against chemical contamination. If it's on your skin, it most likely ends up in your body. This is especially true with laundry detergent because our clothes can be tight, contact moist membranes, rub against the body, as well as become soaked with sweat, further releasing the toxins held within them and being readily absorbed through the skin and into the body.

"For Topical Use Only"—an Oxymoron

There are many products on the market today that are "for topical use only." What this means is that the manufacturer is stating that the product is safe to put on your skin but not safe to eat or use in-vitro. Basically, they are telling you once again that "in small amounts, it is okay," because when it gets on your skin it won't be absorbed as rapidly as it would be had it been ingested. But the reality is, it *is* getting into our bodies, even if we only put it on our skin.

Knowing that the skin is permeable, this makes perfect sense to me. When you apply these chemicals to your skin, they inevitably will end up in your system and left behind for your body to quarantine and eliminate. We continuously, and without realizing it, contaminate our bodies by simply using everyday hygiene products. I firmly believe if you can't put it in your mouth, you shouldn't put it on your skin.

Foods Used as Hygiene Products

I practice this concept in hygiene by using organic fatty oils as hair conditioner/gel and skin moisturizer. Extra virgin organic coconut oil works better than any moisturizer that I have ever tried for dry skin. It creates a clean barrier over the skin to help protect against environmental toxins as well as adding healthy hydration, eliminating dry skin almost immediately. OEVO (organic extra virgin olive (oil)) is another high-quality healthy oil that not only works well for hair and skin but is often used as a carrier for the application of essential oils to the body and also carries healing properties with it.

Not Nearly Enough Scrutiny in Cosmetics

Cosmetics, ironically, get the least amount of scrutiny by the government and therefore contain more known carcinogens than any other category of products regulated by the same administration. We mentioned the existence of sulfates and parabens within most of the hygiene products on the market, but there are an infinite number of compounds being created on a daily basis by the chemists who work for these ambitious cosmetic companies that are potentially very dangerous.

A New Anti-Aging Product Every Day

Seemingly every day you hear about a new breakthrough compound created, claiming the ability to reverse premature aging, which is in reality, mostly caused by the lifelong, continued exposure to these unnatural compounds. Parabens are another group of toxins found in cosmetic products. Some companies discontinued the use of them but later bragged about it in the commercial advertisements, effectively taking focus away from what toxins they do contain.

There are companies boasting about how they don't use hormones in their creation of certain food products, when in reality it's because it's illegal now and no one can do it anyway. This shows us once again that deceit and advertising go hand in hand, and these things especially enrage me because I know people like me are falling for it. These opportunistic advertisers are always putting the spin on these new changes in the industry, trying to convey the idea that they are doing something special, and therefore their brand is superior to the other types available, or worse yet, as good as the organic choices.

Aluminum and Other Heavy Metals

Heavy metals are another problem found not only within our food but within the hygiene and cosmetic products we use today. No, I don't mean mercury or lead, as these are found usually by accident in food. I'm talking about aluminum. Aluminum is a common metal found in some products such as antiperspirants and sun-block lotions.

Also the aluminum found in antiperspirants is directly connected to Alzheimer's, brain disorders, and the abundance of breast cancer today (Robin Wulffson MD, 2012). Adding to this problem was the use of rBST growth hormones in the dairy products throughout the late twentieth century, which accelerated the growth of this cancer at an alarming rate (Robert Cohen, 1997). No longer allowed for use in dairy products as it is a dangerous synthetic hormones for cows, rBST is identical to human growth hormones that end up in the resulting dairy products, having adverse effects on the health of those who consume them. In some European countries, the use of aluminum in hygiene products has been outlawed since the early 1980s.

So it seems you would again have to become a chemist in order to know what is safe and what isn't, especially when it comes to hygiene. For me the answer is simple. If it isn't organic or at least as close to 100 percent natural as possible, it's potentially dangerous to your health. Simplifying your life and your regime with less "stuff" can be a stress-relieving, money-saving, and liberating way to go. Less is more!

Other Cancer-Causing Items Used Every Day

Electromagnetic Fields

Electromagnetic fields (EMF) are fields of energy that are created by electrical devices. EMFs are produced by power lines, electrical wiring, motors, and all types of wireless devices. Power lines have been known to cause different forms of cancer, especially in children, due to this magnetic field. Science has debated this issue for decades.

Like other concepts of health, this has not been proven by studies and is more likely suppressed by those who stand to lose a lot of money if it had to be remedied. Unfortunately, the most in-depth studies have had mixed results. While some find slight correlation between EMF exposure and cancer, others dismiss it by proving that cancer occurred at equal rates in both homes with higher and lower EMF exposure. Personally I think it's impossible to keep track of the actual amount of EMFs that a person is exposed to on a daily basis. Unless, of course, someone was equipped with the correct type of sensing and data-recording equipment for an entire test period, I doubt anyone has spent the money to do so, and if they did, this information would probably be suppressed, as is often the case.

If you keep your cell phone near a computer monitor, when you receive a call, you will notice on the monitor and from the speakers, an interruption causing screen abnormalities, noise, and distortion. This is the EMF from the cell phone causing another electrical device (in this case your computer and monitor) with less intense EMFs to succumb to the more powerful electronic magnetic frequencies of the other device.

Besides being a plumbing contractor, I have been an active musician as well—hauling, lugging, and setting up all kinds of sound equipment, learning how to use these electronics, and what to avoid so you won't have issues. Any signal that is weak, such as a pre-amped signal, needs to be sent to the amplifier through a shielded cable. Because if the signal is weak, it can easily be affected by nearby EMFs, which cause "ugly" frequencies to appear seemingly out of nowhere through the amplifiers and out the speakers.

This is remedied by a protection medium called *shielding*. If I were to use an unshielded cable for an instrument or pre-amp signal, there will be noise interference coming through the amp out the speakers. Another way this can happen is by laying power cables (line voltage) on, near, or around the weak signal "send" cables (weak unamplified signal).

Because we are electrical and have electrical signals used for communication between the bodies' systems, these signals can be interrupted by other stronger EMFs produced by electrical devices in our vicinity. The difference here is we show no signs of this interruption outside the body while it is taking place, unlike the computer or sound gear.

Regardless of the studies, if these EMFs are interrupting electrical signals of other devices, then I think it's obvious that it will interrupt our bodies' electrical signals as well. Any form of interference in the body, especially for an extended period of time, can cause dysfunction, injury, and ultimately health problems.

Microwaved Food

Most people don't believe that heating food in the microwave is not the same as heating food on the stove or in a conventional oven. One example that this is true is the transfusion of human blood to a patient. Before human blood can be transfused, it must be warmed to body temperature. If you were to heat this blood in the microwave, it would *kill* the blood cells and inevitably the recipient.

The most worrisome problem with the use of the microwave oven is the use of plastic containers to heat or to cook the food. Scientists are finding all kinds of carcinogens (dioxins) being released by the plastics, which further contaminate your food when heated (catalyst) by the microwave. Processed and prepackaged food, meant for the microwave, oftentimes come packed in plastic, ready to be heated in the microwave. These foods should be removed from the plastic and placed on a glass or ceramic dish, if you insist on using the microwave.

Do not warm a baby's bottle in a microwave; most of us already know this, but usually for the wrong reasons. So far we have not done any direct studies linking cancers to microwave use, but the release of toxins from plastics in the microwave is true. The blood example is enough for me to not want to use it at all, other than heating water maybe.

Hair Dyes

It is becoming more obvious that hair dyes are chemically laden and dangerous, and as a result can have a contaminating effect on the body. Diaminoanisole and FD&C Red 33 are but two toxins found in hair dyes, which have been directly classified as carcinogens. This concept has been reinforced by many different studies that link hair dyes to such cancers as non-Hodgkin's lymphoma, Hodgkin's disease, and multiple myeloma. Other studies claim that at least 20 percent of non-Hodgkin's lymphoma in women is caused by the use of hair dyes. As usual, there are too many variables to prove what actually causes what, leading us again to the concept of a clean regime. My mother was a beautician and would perform many color and permanent applications throughout her career. After years of being exposed to these chemicals, she became allergic to them and could no longer expose herself to them, as she had developed bad rashes on her hands and arms. With the use of some bag-balm and other natural remedies, she was healed in no time, naturally having stayed away from said chemicals since.

Meats and Eggs Cooked at High Temperatures

Overcooked eggs or burned, charred meat can contain toxic compounds within them. These are some of the same compounds that are found in cigarette smoke. Recent studies suggest a link between these compounds and cancers of the digestive system, mammary glands, oral cavity, and skin.

We all know that fried foods are dangerous due to other types of contamination and high-fat content, but now we have another reason not to eat fried foods. Fried foods are cooked rapidly and at high heat, causing the production of these cancer-causing compounds. We might also need to be careful with grilling and other types of cooking as well. This means raw foods are the best. The problem here is that theoretically it is not safe to consume raw meat (however some people do eat raw meat). I do, however, consume raw (organic) eggs for breakfast and have for years now.

Radiation Sources

Some or most of the radiation we are exposed to comes from medical and dental x-rays. Although necessary in certain medical situations, maybe we should avoid them unless they are absolutely necessary. Chemical agents used to enhance the visibility of these x-rays have been found in the past to cause health problems as well. Today they have new "safe" alternatives to the older versions of these agents, but how long before they find the new one to be dangerous? The rest of the radiation comes from radon gas, which is usually collected in our basements or homes. Radiation comes from other "natural" sources such as the sun. (Fifty thousand people die each year from not getting enough sun).

Mold

Mycotoxin is a toxic compound produced by molds living and growing in your home and environment. These toxins are released by molds into the air of their surroundings. Several kinds of these toxins exist, and they vary with the different species of molds. Most of these toxins produced are hazardous to our health, many of which can be carcinogenic. These types of organisms can infest your home when the right environment is created for them. These toxins can also be found in foods. Eating fresh, local, organic food is always best.

Talc

The mineral talc is used and found in many different products for the house and body. Talc contains within its processed form small particles with the same physical characteristics as asbestos, which can wind up in the lungs through inhalation. It is usually found in small quantities but powdered forms being the most dangerous, as they are easily inhaled. These particles can cause Mesothelioma and other forms of lung cancer, as well as other types of intestinal cancers.

The scary part is some of us use these products almost every day, further adding to the health threat to us all. What's worse is baby powder (use a cornstarch base instead) is a product that is so dangerous, proving we are subject to health dangers as early as birth and before. Numerous cancers may be linked to talcum powder use, but there is no economically viable reason to spend the money to find out.

Pots, Pans, and Plastic Containers

Use only stainless steel, glass, or ceramic cookware and food containers, in, on, or around your food. Plastics vary in chemical makeup, where some plastics are "food grade" and considered safe while others are known to be dangerous. Always choose BPA-free containers, as this is a common contaminate found in bottles, cans, and other packaging and containing products. If you are not sure, don't use it near or around your food to prevent the "spilling" of toxins into it.

Teflon-coated and other nonstick surfaces can release toxins into your food as well. Aluminum foil, cans, and cookware are not to be used around your food as the metals are oftentimes broken down and dissolved into the food, adding more heavy metals to the already possibly contaminated food.

Air "Fresheners"

Air fresheners are made with all kinds of potentially dangerous chemicals within them, which are then aspirated into the air. Needless to say, this is disturbing, especially when you see the commercials with the automatic diffusers that shoot these chemicals right in your face when you walk by. This automated process decides how much of this spray air freshener you will use and when. Some companies boast the use of essential oils within their products, but almost all use some kind of scented oil, which is really just an unnatural scented chemical instead.

The use of therapeutic-grade essential oils as well as live flowers and plants are the best ways to freshen and purify the air in your home, once again, because they are all natural and therefore provide benefits to your health and wellbeing.

Dry Cleaning

Just like the detergents that we use at home, dry-cleaning types of cleansers are made with dangerous chemicals and can also be toxic to the body, if not more toxic. There are alternative, all-natural types of dry cleaners today to choose from.

Although we now have a pretty good idea of where toxins come from and how they get into the body, we must use this knowledge to remain vigilant in preventing our continued exposure to the unnatural. Regardless of whether or not the studies have been done as to the linking of these contaminants to specific disease, it is impossible to know exactly what all these different toxins do to the body, because of the vast array of variables including genetics. Applying the clean regime or the all-natural concepts will give you the ability to make the right decisions when it comes to healthy choices and product safety in the future.

Detoxification

Now that you've learned how our bodies become contaminated and how to test your pH, how do you deal with and eliminate the existing toxins from your body? This is achieved with many different cleansing techniques, used one at a time or simultaneously.

Introduction to Decontamination

In this chapter you will learn of a few different detoxifying techniques that you can do at home. You will use no drugs or unnatural chemicals of any kind during this cleanse. Remember, as always, to ask your doctor, especially if you take medications or are already sick in some way *before you begin!* At the same time, make sure that the decisions you make with your doctor are focused *entirely* on your healing and cure.

Take your time and give yourself a warm-up period, implementing these cleansing techniques slowly. I don't want you to have a bad experience, as this can be such a wonderful experience when done correctly. There are some discomforts that can take place when mistakes are made, and sometimes under normal circumstances, such as constipation, gas, stomachaches, headaches, nausea, tiredness, or even becoming a little irritable. These are side effects of the toxins being drained from the body rapidly, or from existing dysfunction becoming more evident, now that you are asking your body to be more functional. These can sometimes actually be a good sign that your cleansing is working;

it may just mean you need to slow down. If you do this correctly, you will avoid most of these things.

Some more side effects to expect: weight loss is almost guaranteed, if you need to lose any, as most of us do. Because we will be neutralizing fats, they will easily be shed from the body. Also expect a huge increase in energy within four to five days of starting the cleansing period and thereafter if you keep up with your pH.

Two discomforts I experienced, on just a few occasions over nine months, was a headache, which I experienced two weeks into the cleansing and probably a few months later. I blame this indirectly on the alkaline water, as it can drain toxins rapidly, but it's not necessarily the reason. When I experienced these headaches, I would simply stop drinking water until the next day and take a nap.

Hunger will definitely be an issue, not so much on day one, but soon after, especially for most of us who have a poor diet and lots of sugar cravings. Oftentimes these cravings are caused from the starvation of unfavorable microbes like yeast, bacteria, and others that feed on sugars.

If you experience any of these mild discomforts, you should take a break and work through it. If you develop chronic issues, you need to go back and see your doctor, preferably a doctor who knows a little about these techniques as well as your favorite doctor. It is important to include someone who understands what you're doing.

Should I Exercise During a Cleanse?

Exercising is an essential part of a healthy lifestyle; however, I am a firm believer in getting a handle on your pH levels (diet) first. Because so much damage is taking place in our bodies from contamination, it is more important to clean house first in order to facilitate the healing of internal dysfunction we may not be aware of. This is why so many apparently healthy people sustain injury from seemingly mild falls, or seemingly out of nowhere; they are terminally ill with a rare, new disease. Contamination leads to outer physical injury because the body's organs and structure are breaking down from within.

Exercising is not so important during a cleansing; however, we need to sweat in order to eliminate acids. Also we want to move around a bit during the day, as this helps get other things moving as well (the bowels). I suggest a nice twenty-minute walk at any pace each day during this period, even twice a day if you want. If you already train often and with intensity, you should limit your anaerobic activity, as it creates a lot of acid. Focusing more on some less-intense cardiovascular training temporarily, because this allows you to stay active and also helps facilitate sweating. If you do keep exercising during your cleansing, you will need to add as much extra water as possible.

The Need to Sweat

Sweating is imperative to facilitate the elimination of acids. There are a few ways in which this can be done; some are obvious, but if you live in a cold area, it is not always easy. Saunas (dry heat) are the best way to sweat during a cleansing, as it takes no physical activity to cause sweating and does not expose you to contaminants, which are released from water in steam baths. *Do not* use steam as a means of sweat therapy, as the water used for making the steam is usually not purified, and exposing yourself to tap water through the steam medium can be even more dangerous than drinking it. This is true due to the vaporization of contaminants within the water that are inhaled and more rapidly contaminate the body through the lungs as opposed to the skin or intestines.

Other than dry heat saunas, if you live in a warmer area at the right time of year, it can be an easy task to achieve simply by sitting in the heat. And obviously some mild cardiovascular training of some kind can help—going for a brisk walk on the street or treadmill, a few minutes on the elliptical, or stairs, whatever. If your physical condition is such that you cannot go for a twenty-minute walk, due to being confined to a wheelchair or injury, there are exercise programs for you too. Simply moving your arms and raising your legs, if you are able, can burn calories and cause sweating. Again, consult your doctor *before you start* any programs at all!

Water: the Primary Tool in Detoxification

The main item used in detoxification of the body is water, lots of water. Not soda, not fake iced tea, not coffee, not sport drinks, not energy drinks, not flavored waters, not even fruit juice, (with a couple of exceptions), are acceptable for detoxification. Now, since we are using water to decontaminate our bodies, we need to make sure the water that we are drinking is not itself contaminated. Obviously this would be ineffective in cleansing our body, right? So we need to make sure that the water we are using is pure first. Then we would have to see that the pH of the water is neutral at minimum. But preferably we will use the optimum water source mentioned in chapter four.

Acidity and Contamination go Hand in Hand

Acidity and contamination go hand in hand, so to drink acidic water, even if it's not contaminated with carcinogens, can lead to more acidity, as it does not have the ability to neutralize the acids already found in the body. Most of the beverages we drink are acidic, whether it is water or something more, which can further acidify an already acidic body environment. Any drinks that contain sugars, artificial sweeteners, modified sugars, artificial colors, flavors, and preservatives need to be avoided during your cleanse and probably altogether.

No Sugar, Plenty of Hydration

Okay, so we will make the commitment to drink mostly water for the duration of our cleansing. We've said the water should be ionic, alkaline, and pure. We will want to double or even triple the amount of water we *should* drink on a daily basis; this normal amount being one ounce of water per two-to-three pounds of body weight. During our cleansing, we want a 1 to 1.5 ratio or better. For example, if the person weighs 100 pounds, he or she will want to drink fifty to seventy-five ounces of water in order to effectively clean house. A minimum amount should be three quarts per day, with a maximum of two gallons (rare, but I have done it). This will be difficult at first, but we will soon instigate some sweating, which will help. Start slow at first, maybe having a warm-up period for a few days to begin hydration before the full detox begins.

Going without sugars will be a challenge, as most of us are addicted to the vast array of sweeteners out there. You may have a cup of tea early morning or evening, but it should be organic herbal tea, free of caffeine, as these teas are also cleansing. If you absolutely have to have some sweetener, use a teaspoon of honey. This is not going to taste very sweet, but it can help with the taste and cravings. Another way to reduce sugar cravings is to purchase some 70 to 80 percent organic dark chocolate, and eat small pieces when you feel the urge for sweetness.

What Do We Eat During a Cleanse?

It only makes sense if we start with a solution (our body fluid in this case) with a low pH (in the acidic range). As we begin to introduce alkaline minerals/elements, we should see an elevation in pH. This is the reason for staying away from acidic foods during a cleansing. In retrospect, it also makes sense that if we are trying to introduce alkaline elements into a solution (our body fluids) to raise the pH by reaching deep into our bodies' tissues with these alkali, if we were to add acidic elements into our diet during this period, we then neutralize the alkali superficially, before it can reach the acids trapped deep within the cells of the body, which will not facilitate removal of said toxins.

Some examples of acidic foods (even healthy ones) would be any kind of animal proteins or fats (meat, eggs, dairy); sugars and carbohydrates including fruit juice, fruit, breads, and cereals; even some vegetables like squashes are acidic and should be avoided during your cleanse. We said that an acidic body will use fat as a buffer to protect the organs from these dangerous acids. As this is true, animal fat can be highly contaminated. Proteins themselves are made of amino acids, which mean they are made up of acidic elements. Any and all processed foods should also be avoided for now if not altogether.

Healthy forms of chicken, beef, and eggs (in moderation) can be an essential source of complete protein for your diet, so you only need to avoid them during your cleanse. Processed meats of any kind should be avoided, as they are very dangerous to your health; deli meat or any meat shaped like a tube, whether whole (sausage) or sliced (bologna), contain nitrates that cause health problems. Some people get angry with the fact that I do not endorse eating sausage, but it is my opinion that it is dangerous. If you choose to eat these kinds of meats, make sure they are as fresh and natural as possible, and these types of meats should be consumed with even more moderation in mind, more than fresh, pristine, organic, and wild meat choices should be. Any meat should be eaten in balance with the other food choices contained within your diet. Too much meat is typically considered unhealthy.

So you understand when it comes to food choices, you must stay focused on avoiding acidic foods. At the same time you want to make sure that the foods you do eat are free from contamination of *any* kind, again during the cleansing period (and beyond, preferably). You may decide to incorporate some of these concepts later, after your cleansing period, into your regular regime. If you achieve pH balance in your body, you will want to sustain that balance in order to maintain vibrant health. Therefore, it makes sense that continued balancing of the bodies' fluid is the key to the longevity of this pH balance, as well as life and health itself.

Eating Only Alkalizing Foods

You should focus on consuming only alkalizing foods during this time period. These foods consist of most vegetables (green ones being the better ones for alkaline minerals, colored hearty ones more for fiber and moisture), potatoes of all kinds—the whiter the better for a cleanse (don't forget potatoes are vegetables too, but don't eat only potatoes. You can realistically make lightly pan-fried potatoes in canola, with onion for a meal, or in addition to another vegetable or a salad), nuts and nut butters, healthy oils like organic olive (OEVO), peanut, safflower, and canola. Even dried fruits can be used, and let's not forget whole food alkalizing supplements.

Most fruits are alkalizing to the body but still have high-sugar content, and they need to be eaten by themselves on an empty stomach in order to be alkalizing, so we will avoid most fruits for now. Citrus fruits low in sugar such as grapefruits or lemons can be used during a cleansing but still in moderation (unless you are to do a grapefruit cleanse specifically). Because these fruits are acidic (vitamin C) but low in sugar, they have a stronger alkalizing effect on the body but still should be eaten separate from your other foods (wait an hour). Dried fruits are a better choice for your detox, as they are alkaline and provide taste satisfaction and sweetness. These should not be the primary source of food, however, as vegetation will be the primary food source during this time.

Any kind of organic nuts, such as almonds, walnuts, peanuts, pistachios, etc., are all foods that can be eaten, almonds being the best. Keep in mind that the foods that you will eat are going to be mostly *raw*. So when you choose your nuts, choose not only organic ones but raw nuts as well (raw organic almonds are my favorite). This can make it easier for you to prepare your food. Nuts, vegetables, and oils all should be consumed mostly raw, as they are more nutritious in their pristine state (this is true of most foods).

Healthy Oils a Must

Olive oil (OEVO) is one of the best all-around fatty and healing oils. It is a source of mono-unsaturated fats; other sources of mono-unsaturated fats are vegetable, canola, and coconut oil while poly-unsaturated fats can be found in safflower and peanut oils. Any of these oils can be used during the cleansing, preferably raw. These can be used either by themselves or more realistically on your vegetables cold or, if you must, lightly sautéed.

Are Supplements Good for Cleansing?

Besides food, we can and should make use of some whole food, green, antioxidant, herbal, and fibrous supplements. There are many companies selling detox programs and supplements; some of them are good and others not so good. A good indicator is price. If someone is claiming an effective, full-body cleansing program for under $100 US, it may not be what you're looking for. In this world you get what you pay for. If it's cheap, than most likely it's cheap or substandard. However, price should definitely *not* be such a definitive indicator of quality.

Green Supplements a Must

Green supplements are made from dehydrated green vegetation that is concentrated in nutrients. There are many different types, but they are not all created equal. First they should be made of whole, organic plants. No derivatives. The reason is we trust in nature's formulas that consist of all the nutrients found in the plants without alteration or extraction. Next, that they should contain many different types of green vegetation. Some of these plants will be green leafy vegetables; others will be grasses and plants not usually found in the grocery store. Such ingredients should include wheat grass and dandelion.

The best way to judge your greens is to look at them and smell them. They should be very aromatic, having the scent of fresh-cut grass. Next they should be a deep forest green, like fresh spinach. These supplements are procured by juicing the greens, drying the remains, milling them down, and then the original juices are reintroduced in concentrated form. These are then dried again and later ready to use. In a poor-quality green supplement, there is usually more of the dehydrated and juiced leftovers contained in them and less (if any) of the concentrated juices placed back in them, which is where the nutrients are found. These would not have the right ratio of juice-to-fiber and therefore look different. This is obvious, as the contents will be more gray than green. Quality greens should give the physical appearance of fresh-cut vegetation.

Neutralizing Free Radicals

Next is a whole food antioxidant formula consisting of organic, dried, dehydrated, and antioxidant-rich fruits. Most of us know that berries possess most of the antioxidant capabilities among foods. We see commercials about fruit juices made with pomegranate, grapes, and cranberries, etc., boasting high antioxidant content. Citrus-type fruits contain antioxidants as well, so you might see some of these types of fruit added to the formulas as well.

Are You Getting Enough Fiber?

Fiber is so important to good health. Soluble and insoluble fibers are necessary for everyday health and even more important during our cleansing. These are the substances that help physically clean the intestines as well as the individual cells of the entire body. Insoluble fibers do not dissolve into small pieces and help sweep through the colon, effectively eliminating toxins. Soluble fiber will dissolve in water that can actually help structure the fluid in the body, which helps facilitate cellular cleansing.

There are many different types of fiber supplements out there, but I believe, as usual, the more natural ones are better. I use psyllium fiber for an insoluble version. There are a few different sources of cleansing supplement type fibers that I have tried and found to be effective, but in most cases, the ones that need to be mixed with water prior to consuming are typically the best.

Detoxifying Herbal Supplements

Next are your herbal supplements. There are thousands of plants and herbs in the world. The correct formulas for detoxifying different parts of the body have been discovered through their uses throughout history, as well as from more modern studies. This is where the chemistry really takes place; things are happening that we are unaware of (but know are working because we can feel it) but are taking place. This is where the love of our Creator manifests itself through the use of these tools, which were left behind by Him for us.

Fungus, Yeast, Microbes, and Parasites

Besides chemical contamination, what about microbial, fungal, and parasitic contamination? Most people don't consider this possible, as it is typically not heard of often on the news or other TV programs. Nor do you see any of these anti-parasitic drugs advertised on television either. These are all examples of contaminations that take place in the body, probably more often than we realize. When our digestive systems become impacted with putrefying fecal matter and we continue to consume questionable food, this sets the stage for yeasts, fungus, and parasitic infestation (imbalance) within the colon and beyond.

There are a few types of detoxification tools for this kind of infection. One is to use an organic tincture made with oregano and other types of herbs. These herbs are toxic to the microbes and parasites but do not harm us! That's the beauty of nature at work. Another technique is the use of colloidal silver. Colloidal means small enough to pass through the cell wall. Silver in this case refers to the element silver, which is broken down to colloidal size pieces and suspended in distilled or purified water.

Silver also works on bacterial and viral infections as well. This is achieved not by being toxic to the microbes but by being friendly. Friendly? These microbes, like a hermit crab looking for a shell, attach themselves to the metal, only to be flushed out of the body during normal evacuations. This is beneficial, because unlike antibiotics this technique does not "hurt" the microbes, which does not promote the evolution of stronger microbial DNA, which inevitably leads to more deadly types of microbes, as we saw with E. coli in cows. Keep in mind the dosing directions on the container as there are people out there who seriously overuse colloidal silver and have had some weird side effects (the grey woman in Guinness). I have, however, used it successfully several times over the past few years for cleansing and illness prevention without any negatives.

What about the Good Bacteria?

You may not be aware, but the fact is that you need to replenish the "good" bacteria (probiotics) into the intestines during and after using antibiotics, colloidal silver, and other colon cleansers. The reason should be obvious, as the cleansing action removes all microbial infestation—the good bacteria as well as the undesirable ones. Our bodies, due to the processing and preserving of food, are already low on favorable bacteria and probably should be replenished on a regular basis, regardless of microbial cleansing. These bacteria were found in our food for thousands of years, but due to the use of chemicals that kill bacteria during food production and processing, these levels are low or non-existent today.

Many Probiotic Sources to Choose From

Probiotics are different strains of bacteria that are beneficial to the body's defenses and digestive system. We and the bacteria have evolved together, like a clownfish to an anemone, and have developed a harmonious relationship together over thousands of years. These bacteria help with digestion and absorption of nutrients. At the same time, they help us fight off infection by helping with pH balance and killing off foreign, unfavorable bacteria before they have a chance to overwhelm the body.

There are many products on the market claiming to have the best formulas or even their own patented versions of these bacteria. Again, I only trust in what's been around for thousands of years and do not agree with man-altered substances. Besides the unnatural, there are other factors to consider when choosing a pro-biotic supplement. One is dosage. Are there enough bacteria within each dose to be effective? If there *is* a high dose, are they alive when you acquire and consume them? When cleansing, you should use a high-dose formula.

There are types of bacteria that can live without refrigeration as well as ones that cannot. In some cases, non-refrigerated is a better choice, as they are less fragile and can be taken with you. Bacteria requiring refrigeration can be a very good choice as well. Either way you need to be sure that they are from viable sources. There are manufacturers that guarantee viability; these companies usually sell to health practitioners, so you could call them medicinal-grade bacteria. Yogurts are not usually a good enough source of these bacteria because they do not contain enough bacteria to be therapeutic. I used both refrigerated types as well as the non-refrigerated. Both types were purchased from a reliable source that I will share with you on my website.

Digestive Enzymes Digestive Aids

Next are digestive enzyme supplements. These are substances that are used to break down the foods that we consume. In a perfect world, our digestive systems would be functioning properly, and there would be no need to add these digestive aids. The reason we will use these is not only to help digest the foods that you will be consuming during your cleansing and perhaps beyond but to help rid the body of putrefying foods that are currently stuck in the digestive system. *Raw*, organic apple cider vinegar can and will be used in the example programs in the next chapter as a digestive aid, as well as an overall cleansing, alkalizing agent.

Continuing on, you need to incorporate some whole body detoxification herbal supplements. These are used typically, if not already within the colon cleanse, along with the colon cleanse. Later would be an acid drainage-type supplement; these are usually some form of diuretic (organic of course!) used to help drain acids by inducing more urine evacuations, which reinforces that a lot of water is necessary during and after the cleansing.

So now we understand some of the components used in the different cleansing programs, next we need to put together a schedule of when and how to use these products. In the next chapter, you will discover many different techniques, from the most intense to the least. You will need some or all of the components mentioned prior and listed below for your cleansing program, depending which techniques you should choose to use.

Supplements

Distilled water

pH water supplements (minerals for water)

Greens Complex

Antioxidant Complex

Fiber supplements

Acid drainage

Herbal Detox

Microbial detox agent tinctures and colloidal silver

Pro-biotics

Digestive enzymes

Organic Food

Potatoes

Broccoli, zucchini, cauliflower, carrots

Spring mix, spinach, cucumbers, tomatoes

Olives (oil cured)

Raw organic apple cider vinegar

Honey, 100 percent pure

Almonds

Raisins

Lemons

Olive oil

Here Are Some More Alkalizing Foods That Can Be Used

Alkaline:

Asparagus, barley, grass

Bamboo shoot, beets

Broccoli, Brussels sprouts

Cabbage, carrot

Cauliflower, celery

Collard greens, cucumber

Eggplant, garlic

Green beans, green olives

Green peas, kale

Kelp, lettuce

Mushrooms, mustard greens

Onions, parsley

Parsnips, peas

Peppers, potato

Pumpkin, radishes

Sea veggies, spinach

Sprouts, sweet potatoes

Tomatoes, watercress

Wild greens

Healthy Acidic Foods Your Body Needs Acids Too. It Just Needs the Right Ones; However, You Will Avoid Them during Your Cleansing

Artichoke

Black olives (unless they are oil-cured)

Corn

Mushrooms

Pickles

Sauerkraut

Squash

Detoxification How-To

In this chapter, I will talk about the different techniques for cleansing the body, starting with the most intensive program, and later discussing the less intensive or less involved ones. The most intensive program, addressing a more heavily acidic system, shall be detoxifying to all the body's systems as well as provide an increase in overall pH balance. People who are less acidic, but are new to some of the concepts in this book, can choose to try some of the less intensive means of cleansing. You need to be honest with yourself as to how toxic your body might be by taking a good look at lifestyle, possible exposures, *and* by testing your overall pH as described in chapter three.

As Always, Ask Your Doctor

As *always*, you'll need to check with your licensed health professional before starting *any* detox program. This is especially true if you are ill and taking medications of any kind, due to possible interactions. If you take multiple medications on a daily basis (which is far from uncommon today), your doctor most likely will suggest omitting the use of herbal products because they do not require FDA regulation. Most doctors do not know enough about these types of medicinal substances. Also, they cannot tell you to stop taking your current prescriptions, as there are liability issues to consider.

If you are not ill and do not take any medications of any kind, you still need to seek the advice of a licensed healthcare professional who is well versed in these areas. Professionals to consider might be a licensed naturopath, nutritionist, or other holistic professional found in wellness centers and on their own. "Holistic" no longer means that they are self-proclaimed healers, or worse, some kind of snake oil salesman but are licensed healthcare professionals who offer many different types of alternative therapies.

How to determine what cleansing program to use for your situation, again, is based on your toxicity level, which is represented by your overall pH of your intracellular fluid. If your pH is at or above a reading of 6.5, then you have only a slight deviance in optimum pH levels and might decide that a less intensive program or even an instant and permanent change in diet would be enough. A pH level of 6.0 to 6.5 might call for a somewhat more intense program. If you have a pH level that is below 5.9 or worse, then the more or even the most intensive program should be used, at least for your first cleanse, again, only after talking to your licensed healthcare practitioner.

Intensive Detoxification Program Start

The following is an intensive example of a cleansing or detoxification program. This program is best started on a Friday, as it will give you the weekend for the hardest days. There are unlimited variables that can be done using the same ingredients. Some of these variables include duration of cleansing period. For an intensive cleansing, you must cleanse for at least seven days, especially if you have a very acidic system, as most people today do. Other variables would be the difference in the ratio of fresh food to supplements (the types of foods that you choose will vary but must conform to the alkaline food list), how many times a day you eat food or take supplements, and how much water you drink.

Some people will be able to drink more water and should if they can, but we will represent this as a minimum of one ounce of water per two pounds of body weight per day, or three quarts is better if you can, unless the previous is more. You can choose to eat different vegetables as long as you get some heavy, leafy greens and some higher volume fibrous ones as well. This will allow you to customize your detox and future diet plan. Keep in mind you need to stick to *only* certified organic food choices during the cleansing program.

Do *You* Need a Warm-Up?

A warm-up period is usually required, as most people have an impacted colon and need to take some extra time and start gradually. I recommend starting with cleaning up your diet (eating only organic foods) and add the consumption of the recommended amount of daily water to your regime for an entire week. So this would mean to switch from your regular food choices to better quality organic ones and drink a lot of good, quality water. If you have problems being irregular, you should see an improvement in this area. If you do not see an improvement, you can do the following for another week.

A Regularity *and* Overall Healthy Technique

Upon waking: in an eight to twelve-ounce glass, mix one to two tablespoons of raw, organic, apple-cider vinegar, along with one to two tablespoons of pure honey (local is best). Mix thoroughly and drink immediately before breakfast. The vinegar can be reduced to one tablespoon if two is too much; however, if you first drink four ounces of water mixed with one level teaspoon of baking soda (sodium bicarbonate), this will coat your stomach lining, protecting it from the added acids (vinegar). This soda can be used as a temporary relief of heartburn or indigestion from overeating or nervous stomach as well. Consume this cider vinegar drink directly before dinnertime. Take a high dosage of a viable form of probiotics immediately after dinner. Do this all the while continuing to consume the recommended amount of healthy water per day and choosing better quality, organic food choices. This warm-up period can be used as a mild cleansing.

Be sure not to take any fiber supplements if you have major chronic constipation. You will need to get your bowels moving before you add fiber supplements in order to avoid pain and or discomfort within the abdomen. If you have chronic constipation, you should see your doctor or healthcare practitioner about this problem and maybe consider the use of colon hydrotherapy.

It's Time to Add Some Supplements

Next is to begin to use some of the other supplements, introducing them slowly, starting with half-doses to prevent an undesirable effect. Continue to use the cider drink first thing in the morning. Follow this immediately with a serving of greens, antioxidants, minerals, fibers, and enzymes. Some of the previously mentioned supplements can be obtained in capsule form as well as powder. However, most of the fiber supplements require mixing with water in order to consume, as they will bind you up without it, leading to gas and bloating, and will not work properly without the added water. The idea is to hydrate the digestive system that will rejuvenate it and get it moving at a healthier rate. This is another reason for drinking an ample amount of water daily on a regular basis.

This technique can be done for a week, if you want, without implementing the vegan diet or alkaline foods-only portion of the cleansing period, which is the hardest part. This technique takes longer but will ensure a pleasurable experience in the end. If you're anxious to get started, you can reduce the warm-up time periods.

Take It to the Next Level

Time to kick it into high gear! Continue to use the cider drink and the supplements previously mentioned in the morning. After one hour, take a dosage of the anti-microbial cleansing agent (colloidal silver or organic tincture) colon cleanser with fiber, as well as your herbal decontaminating complexes, remembering to drink a lot of water before, with, and after this step. One to one and a half hours later, it's time to replace the good bacteria that were swept away by the fiber and microbial cleansing agents. We will achieve this with a serving of our high-dose viable pro-biotics at the same time; take some of your acid drainage (natural diuretic i.e., cranberries) supplement. Again, follow each step with plenty of water.

In another hour or so, it's time to eat. It's better to drink a good amount of water before you eat rather than after. A giant salad with many different leafy vegetables, covered with some olive oil and a hint of lemon juice or cider vinegar, topped with some sliced almonds or sunflower seeds will do just fine. Or even just a handful of almonds and raisins are okay too. If you have time, baked potatoes with sautéed spinach, broccoli, and carrots is tasty and healthy as well. I will have more diet and recipe ideas for you on our website.

In two hours, it's time to repeat this cycle again. This can be done up to three times a day. You can decide to eat more food and take fewer supplements or vice versa, but you should not cycle through the supplements more than three times a day. Remember, you must end the supplement cycle with pro-biotics every time. You can eat as much as you want, as often as you want, as long as you consume mostly vegetables, raw being best, remembering to refrain from meat, animal fats, sugars, or other acidic foods.

This cleansing is broken down into three segments with at least an hour between them. First is eating, whether it is food or supplements. Next is cleansing; this is when we take colon and whole body detoxifying agents. And third is replenishing, this consisting of the pro-biotics and the diuretics if used. Food should be consumed separate from the colon cleanse and pro-biotics.

My Cleansing Program Customization

The first time I did this program, I used the cider drink and supplements in the morning starting with the cider drink, followed by the food/supplement portion of the cleansing, followed two hours later by the colon cleansing and fiber, as always drinking a ton of water with each step, following the cleansers with the pro-biotics and diuretics (acid drainage) an hour later. During the rest of the day, I ate several servings of carrots, cucumbers, tomatoes, salad with olive oil, almonds, and water during the work day. At dinnertime I would make baked potatoes, sautéed broccoli, cauliflower, baby spinach, and zucchini in canola oil and sometimes have another salad. To deal with the sugar cravings, I would eat small bites of organic 70 percent dark chocolate (I have a really big sweet tooth).

I did this for a week or two. When I was done with my more intense cleanse, I later began adding a small, quality meat product to my dinner. So my cleansing diet was altered slightly and became my regular diet. This addition of protein had been introduced after a couple of weeks of cleansing with the more intensive vegan diet and should not be done before you have completed at least one week of intensive cleansing. After you have completed a total of four weeks minimum, including your warm-up period, you are done! Time to check your pH again! You should see a drastic increase in your levels.

It's recommended that you continue to use the cider drink now and then for energy, alkalizing properties, and immune boosts. The supplements used in this program are good to have on hand and can be used to do just that: supplement nutrients that you should get from your regular diet of food but occasionally don't due to hectic lifestyle. Greens, minerals, fiber, pro-biotics, and antioxidant formulas are examples of everyday supplements that can be used on a semi-regular basis.

Obviously we are busy, and it's not always easy to consume the right foods at the right time, each day, consistently. But it is recommended that you continue the cleansing diet with the addition of fruits, moderate sugar use, and four to six ounces of quality meat product a few times a week. Make this your regular diet.

Cheating now and then once your body is clean (not during the cleanse) is okay because your body can deal with a little bit of the unnatural now and then, as long as you continue to give it the tools and opportunity to keep up with the mess; however, if you eat clean for an extended period of time, when you do eat crappy food, you will notice the difference in taste (especially saltiness) and how it makes you feel right away.

Other Cleansing Techniques to Try

Next are some examples of cleansing regimes that are variations of the previous and might not require as many supplements to practice. In the first example, you will do basically the same regime as the first without some of the supplements. Clean water; raw, organic apple cider vinegar; pro-biotics; and plenty of organic foods are a must.

This next version of the original full-body cleanse is to start with the cider drink again in the morning, followed by a serving of greens, antioxidants, minerals, enzymes, and fiber. A smoothie of some kind will allow you to add these to your morning meal. Eat a clean diet similar to your original but customize it to adapt some of these new healthy concepts we have learned; in addition, refrain from eating meat temporarily. Lots of water is a must, as always, because no cleansing program works without it. Pro-biotics after a well-balanced dinner will complete this cleanse for the day. This can be a regular diet for some or a short-term cleanse for others.

Vegetables Used to Keep the Body Clean

Stick to a vegetarian diet (all food except meat) as best you can during the day for all cleanses, making sure to consume a large amount of vegetables and water, adding some healthy oils (2 tbsp.) into your diet a few times a day. Raw nuts also provide the good oils into your diet. For supper, have a well-balanced meal consisting of a protein source (four ounces boneless chicken breast), an organic grain (1/3 cup basmati brown rice), and a generous portion of steamed vegetables. Choose healthy snacks like fruits, nuts, dark chocolate (70 percent or better), and nut butters on whole grains as well.

Another version of a less intense cleansing is achieved by starting your day with the cider drink then followed shortly by a fruit smoothie with a fiber supplement added. Make sure to use all-natural ingredients, whole, organic fruits mixed with your reliable water. Honey blue agave and maple syrup are the healthiest forms of sweetener, but there are other stevia-based ones and natural (organic) forms of cane juice or sugar. If you feel you need to add sweetness, keep in mind that too much sugar, even organic kinds, are bad for you due to their acidifying effects and resulting blood sugar spike. The best forms of sweetener again are honey, maple syrup, and blue agave. When you do eat sweets, you should have them close to your dinner and not on an empty stomach. By eating proteins and/or complex carbohydrates before or with the high-sugar foods, it will help anchor the sugars so they don't digest too fast and cause blood sugar elevation to happen too rapidly. Keep in mind most breakfast foods that don't contain eggs or meat are made mostly of simple sugars. This is a big problem today with most diets. Consuming mostly sugar and caffeine in the morning on an empty stomach causes consistent blood-sugar spikes, which further leads to more acidification of the body and strain on the pancreas.

These secondary variations to the first, most intense cleanse are not too far from what a healthy diet should be on a regular basis, except that you are limiting your meat consumption to once a day and red meat to twice a week. This is a good practice to follow anyway, but some people believe proteins in the morning are good for maintaining healthy blood sugar. As a body builder, I have always eaten protein in the morning during training periods (mostly eggs). Eggs are a healthier form of protein than any fleshy meat, but they still slow down your digestive system like other proteins. This is why we will refrain from eggs and meat during the colon cleanses. You want to get your digestive system moving fast, at least temporarily. This is how you effectively clean the colon.

High-mercury fish will also be omitted during the cleansing period as well and later limited to a six-ounce portion once a week. Sardines and herring are better choices because you don't have to limit yourself to a six-ounce portion once a week that contains more omega-3 than deep ocean fish. Don't forget that you will not be drinking any other beverages other than water except for herbal teas in moderation. You should also keep in mind that you want to avoid anything that is, again, unnatural. Never underestimate the importance of the correct water source and to drink enough of it.

Other Less-Intensive Cleansing Techniques

From here I will describe some cleansing techniques you can add to your current regime but aren't considered full-body, organ-specific, or complete-cleansing programs. One example of this is to add the cider drink right before you eat in the morning and evening, as this will have an overall cleansing, energizing, and alkalizing effect. In addition, choosing healthier food choices and consuming more hydrating foods like fruits and vegetables will also have a cleansing effect. This compared to a diet that doesn't include these types of food can be a complete turnaround in how you feel. Don't forget that lots and lots of water is a must in all cleansing programs and beyond!

Fasting Can Be an Effective Cleansing Tool

Another example is a fasting-type cleanse that uses water and fruit to hydrate and flush the body. One or two days of eating grapefruits and/or lemons and drinking a large volume of water is an effective way to detoxify the body quickly. The citrus fruits with *low* sugar and high citric acid are the only effective types, as high-sugar content will prevent effective cleansing. These types of cleanses should not be used for more than two days and are superficial compared to the more intensive ones.

Another simple, quick cleanse can be to use the cider drink a few times a day while eating nothing but organic apples on the same day. This cleanse should be done for a day or two only; apples are good, but we need more variety in our diet after a while.

I don't advise mixing the citrus-fruit cleanses with the apple-fruit cleanses, as it can lead to indigestion. Apples and grapefruits don't mix well, at least not for me. Or you could simply fast for a whole day, all the while drinking tons of water, as this will be necessary to cleanse yourself effectively. Sometimes giving our digestive systems a rest can make a big difference.

If you spend some time looking into the supplements and detoxification programs available to you, they can give you new ideas for cleansing techniques as well. If you choose to buy a complete cleansing program from a reputable company, you should follow their instructions for doing so. You can and should always add the cider drink (or other means of consuming raw organic apple cider vinegar), fiber, and probiotics to any cleansing program. And no matter what anyone says, lots of clean, healthy water is a must!

Here is a summary of your different cleansing regimes in the order that they are presented in this chapter.

Most Intense Cleansing Program

Warm up first. Add water for a week, and maybe water and the cider drink for another week, and then begin the following on week three:

- Have cider drink in the morning with 16 oz water minimum. Take greens, antioxidants, fibers, enzymes, and alkaline minerals.

- Drink more water. Wait 1 to 1-1/2 hours. Then, with a glass of water, take colon cleanser, herbal detox, and anti-microbial complexes.

- Drink more water. Wait about an hour. Then, with a glass of water, take probiotics and your acid drainage supplement.

- Drink more water. Wait 1 hour. Then drink a glass of water.

- Eat lunch: Large salad including lots of leaves, cucumbers, tomatoes, almond slices, covered with 2 tbsp. of olive oil and a hint of cider vinegar.

- Drink a glass of water, and wait two hours.

Do this up to three times a day. If you only do this once, you'll have to add more meals to your diet.

First Variation

- Have a cider drink in the morning.

- Smoothie: 16 oz water, banana, two strawberries, greens, minerals fiber, and enzymes, 1/4 cup rolled oats, and honey. Blend and drink. Wait 1/2 hour.

- Drink a glass of water; wait two hours.

- Drink a glass of water.

- Eat lunch (vegetarian).

- Drink a glass of water; wait two hours

- Drink a glass of water

- Have a snack (alkalizing)

- Drink a glass of water; wait two hours

- Drink a glass of water

- Eat a balanced dinner (lots of vegetables)

- Take probiotics

Second Variation

- In the morning, have a cider drink.

- Smoothie same as above or add 2 egg whites.

- After 1/2 hour, drink a glass of water.

- Wait two hours after drinking smoothie before eating again. Drink a glass of water each time before you eat. Eat as cleanly as possible, choosing healthy food based on what you have learned. The rest of the cleansings are simple yet effective for a quick detoxification.

Other Decontamination Techniques

Besides using food, herbs, and supplements, there are other ways to cleanse the body. Most of these require going to visit a professional to obtain these services. Some techniques are more intense than others. They vary in cost and availability, and some are easier than others to perform or take part in.

Ions Prove Beneficial to the Body Again

One way that I have tried with pleasing results is an ionic hydrotherapy cleanse. This therapy is a sophisticated yet simple system that works with the body's natural means of cleansing. Your feet are placed in a basin of water (conductor) with a special device called an array placed between them. The array produces charged ions that flow through your body acting like a magnet, pulling toxins and heavy metals from the body. The toxins exit your body through the pores in your feet via osmosis. This therapy is a safe, effective, and gentle means of cleansing the body, reducing the burden on organs from heavy metals and other toxins, which significantly reduces the possibility of injury. The therapy takes from one half to one hour in duration; within the first five to ten minutes, you can see the elemental toxins being pulled from the body and trapped into the water. Different colors represent different types of toxins.

Another Use for Coffee, or Is It?

Another means of cleansing the body is to get a colonic. Although the thought sounds strange and uncomfortable, it can be a very effective way of cleansing the lower digestive system. Since most contamination starts in the colon, to begin here is not a bad idea. Getting multiple colonics over a short detoxifying period will make the cleansing experience that much more effective and satisfying.

Some people need to do this first because they cannot get their bowels moving at a normal rate in order to effectively cleanse. If you have difficulty doing so, you should see a licensed health care practitioner about your issue.

Exterior Mechanical Manipulation of Toxins

Deep-tissue, hot-stone, Swedish, and other forms of massage not only relieve stress and cause relaxation but mechanically help release toxins from the body's tissues. As always, you need to drink a lot of healthy water before and immediately following any type of massage. This is a situation where consuming purified water for the remains of the day can be healthy by effectively removing the toxins produced after a massage (this works better when you have strong mineral stores).

A Little Sanding Never Hurt Anybody

Salt, sugar, oatmeal, mineral, and other types of full body exfoliation will address decontamination of the body's largest organ: the skin. If you engage in such therapies, it is important that all of the components used are of the highest quality and are completely all natural. This includes the water involved.

Contaminated water is not welcome in any case, especially when it's to be used for therapeutic purposes. Even if this water is going to be used simply to rinse exfoliation mediums from the skin, it should still be purified. Make sure the spa that you patronize for these therapeutic services has a very clean if not purified water source for their hydrotherapy services.

Relaxing Facial and Shoulder Massage

Facials can help with detoxifying the skin of the face, which tends to be one of the main focuses today and probably forever. Facials can be a very pleasurable experience, as they often consist of a relaxing shoulder, neck, and head massage. Using oils, herbs, and other mediums, your skin is cleansed mechanically and chemically. These techniques often leave you with a healthy glow and a feeling of youthfulness.

The Cleansing Capabilities of Plants

The diffusion, application, and ingestion of essential oils, which are derived from the smart distillation of plant matter, are a very effective way to cure what ails you and help decontaminate the body. Aromatherapy has been used for thousands of years. Forgotten over the centuries, cultures of all denominations have used essential oils for stress reduction, spiritual uplifting, meditation, focus, and chronic health conditions, as well as cleaning themselves and their homes. Essential oils can also effectively be used for eliminating microbial infestations of *all* kinds. You will learn that these oils have unique detoxifying capabilities and more in the chapter titled "Essential Oils."

Can Water Therapy Clean and Heal?

Hydrotherapy is vaguely defined as the external application of water to the body in any form for therapeutic purposes. Obviously the main component is water; once again it is impossible to effectively decontaminate the body with these techniques if the water itself is toxic.

Some of these might be familiar to you in the form of a whirlpool or hot tub. This does not mean that a public hot tub or even your own hot tub is safe. It must be a fill and drain type whirlpool, and it must be filled with purified or very clean water of some kind. Hot tubs, swimming pools, and whirlpools are all potentially dangerous as they are filled with chemically laden water, which does not qualify as therapeutic. There is a new type of filtration system for pools and spas that use salt water for treatment instead of chlorine, which is very safe in comparison.

If you have an effective, whole-house water filtration system in your home that is well maintained, you will have clean water available to use therapeutically; however, it should not be used as a source of drinking water. If you do not have a filter, and the water you have available to you has chlorine in it (municipal), you can get a showerhead filter. This will give your hot showers a therapeutic effect and cleanse the body, without the effects of chlorine on your hair, skin, and subsequently your internal organs.

Heat It up and Get Sweating

Sweating is one of the three ways that the body eliminates acids. Exhaling and urinating are the other two ways this is achieved. Getting your body to sweat on a regular basis will help with the elimination of toxins. There are a few ways that you can cause sweat.

Exercising with enough intensity for an ample duration of time will facilitate the sweating process. Besides causing you to sweat, the use of resistance training can actually squeeze the toxins from the muscle and surrounding tissues, eliminating them more efficiently through sweat. This is the best way as exercise is essential to optimum health anyway. Another means of causing sweating is to sit in a dry heat sauna. Don't forget; if you're going to instigate some heavy sweating, you must drink a lot of water.

Don't forget that we should avoid strenuous exercise while we are doing a deep chemical cleanse of the body. Only after your pH is balanced should you begin or restart a regular exercise program. This is done as an everyday cleanse, which should be part of your regular lifestyle.

Dry Heat Is Usually the Safest

Dry heat is the safest form of heat therapy and works well to instigate sweating without a lot of effort. Steam heat can be very good as well but falls under the umbrella of hydrotherapy, requiring pure water. The natural environment can provide you with hot enough temperatures at the right time of year. As a plumbing and HVAC contractor, I spend a lot of time in attics, which can provide a nice makeshift sauna. When it's hot enough, you don't need the attic. Sometimes your own living room without the air conditioning on will do. Or you could sit outside for a few hours during the summer, instead of just sitting in the AC.

Tanning Equipment to Cleanse the Body

Getting enough sun is critical to the production of vitamins in the body. Most of us don't get enough sun, as we have become more sedentary and stuck indoors. When the production of vitamins is accomplished efficiently, this will greatly improve your body's functions and immune system. There are new tanning/light therapy beds that are equipped with special bulbs that emit just the right amount of UVB, infrared, red, and blue light, which are the four colors of the beneficial vitamin-producing light spectrum.

At the same time, it is important to get some natural sunlight each day. This does not mean you should be out in the sunlight all day with no clothes on. Twenty minutes of direct or sixty minutes of indirect sunlight is a happy medium between the previous and none. Genetics plays a role here. Some skin types can handle more sun than others.

Add Living Plants to Your Home

Introducing living plants in your home can add to your detoxification and clean regime program by cleansing the air and adding oxygen to your environment. Plants also consume the acidic waste product CO_2 and produce oxygen (isn't nature awesome?).

Mechanical air purifiers are beneficial to good health as well. Let's face it. If you clean the toxins out of the air that you are breathing, the body will sustain less exposure to them, which is a pre-emptive way of cleansing the body. Vacuuming with a quality machine that is equipped with a HEPA filter can also help with not only pulling these impurities out of the air but removing them from the environment after they have settled on the floor. This action without the use of a HEPA filter will simply redistribute these toxins back into the air.

Yoga and stretching can help with cleansing the body as well. Stretching the muscles not only helps lengthen and strengthen them, but it helps squeeze out the toxins from the muscle and joint tissues as well. Yoga will not only facilitate stretching but help open circulation and electrical systems, providing more efficient body system operations. An efficient body will be able to cleanse itself more readily and easily.

There are many other forms of cleansing the body out there, but these are the ones I am familiar with and have tried. If you are ill, you should seek the assistance of a licensed healthcare professional before using any of the methods described in this book or elsewhere. Also make sure that the professionals that offer these techniques are fully licensed and reputable for their profession.

Essential Oils

Essential oils go hand in hand with the concept of using and consuming plant life for optimum health, with some major differences. Essential oils come from plants, leaves, wood, and bark. They are concentrated versions of the aromatic, oily portion of the plant's lifeblood. They are derived through the smart distillation of these different forms of vegetation.

Medicine Derived through the Distillation of Plants

During the distillation process, the plant's "blood" is vaporized, condensed, and separated into three parts. First is the water-based portion of the distilling. Second is the alcohol-based portion of the resulting solution, and finally the oily part. This "blood" is referred to as oleo-gum-resin. This term recognizes the three different types of substances held within the plant's life sustaining fluids.

These three types of liquids are separated after recapturing the vapors created by the steam distillation. The alcohol portion is sometimes used to make tinctures like microbial cleansers, while the water-based portions are called hydrosols, are often used for hydrotherapy techniques. Finally the oily parts are the essential oils. All parts are safe and healthy to use, but the oils are extra special indeed, because of the unique compounds that they possess (David Stewart, 2009).

Cleansing Compounds Cannot Be Recreated by Man

The compounds found within these oils have some highly unique properties. They differ greatly from any manmade compounds. In that they have an AMU (atomic molecular unit) smaller than any other compound in the chemical manufacturing world. The reason this is favorable is that they are able to pass through the blood-brain barrier, delivering their therapeutic effects almost instantly by entering the bloodstream through the nose (David Stewart, 2009).

Aromatherapy: More Than We Realize

Oils can be used in a few ways; you can ingest them, they can be rubbed on the skin in almost any area of the body, or these benefits can be achieved by simply inhaling these oils. That's right, I'm referring to aromatherapy. For thousands of years, man has used essential oils for all types of health and hygiene purposes, such as cleansing themselves, their homes, and their goods. They were also used for fighting microbial infestation and preserving the dead.

Ancient Secrets of Health and Longevity Lost

Using essential oils was commonplace in the homes and lives of people in the past, but these secrets have been lost over the last few hundred years. Some secrets are making a comeback due to the great information age that we live in. Most of us have heard of aromatherapy, but do we really understand what is happening? Yes, these aromas give you different sensations like relaxation, stress reduction, spiritual uplifting, and mood enhancement, but most of us do not understand how powerful these substances really are at providing healing of the body's deficiencies.

The More the Healthier: Mixing Oils

Oils can be used by themselves or mixed together to work in perfect harmony. Some oils can be applied directly to the skin, while others need to be mixed with carrier oil *before* being applied. Carrier oil is non-aromatic, fatty oil such as olive, walnut, almond, and others. These carriers help reduce the rate of absorption of the essential (aromatic) oils in order to prevent discomfort of the applied area. If you have sensitive skin, you can mix all of your essential oils with a carrier. These carrier oils should be of the organic, virgin qualities, as contamination can cause your essential oils to be dangerous instead of healthy (David Stewart, 2009).

Natural Compounds Win Again

Man has not been able to achieve this characteristic of breaking the blood-brain barrier so far, even in the medical world. This is due to a protection system installed at this junction, put there by our Creator, to protect us from toxins from the air and in our blood. Nature, however, does have the capability to pass through this barrier with its unique carbon-based compounds. These compounds found within the essential oils gratefully and as expected have this ability because they are natural (put there by our Creator) and have healing abilities (David Stewart, 2009).

These compounds are called turpenes and are carbon based. These turpenes have the ability to provide deep cleansing on many levels. Monoturpenes and sesquiterpenes along with phenyl-propanoids give these oils the ability to clean the cell receptors, erase and deprogram false or corrupt information within the cell memory, and reprogram cellular memory with the proper information, which now is being received from the other cells of the body (David Stewart, 2009).

Your cells contain an area within them used to store information. This is not unlike a computer with a hard drive containing valuable information. This area within the cell is called cellular memory. Just like the data on a hard drive, the data stored within the cell memory can become corrupt. This can be corrected by the unique compounds found in these essential oils, facilitating a deep cleansing down at the cellular level.

Lies and Deceit at a Cellular Level

When cellular contamination is high because the cell receptors become blocked inhibiting the flow of oxygen, nutrition, and electricity, cellular mutation can take place. This electricity is information transmitted by the body, which is then received in order to keep the individual cells up to date on current events. When the information cannot be properly transmitted, the individual cell will not have the updated information and therefore can be acting on lies or false information. These compounds have the ability to first remove the blockage of elemental contamination from the cell receptors, allowing the flow of electrical signals (information) back into the cell, as well as oxygen, nutrients, and other types of chemical signals. From here these compounds act like the format button on your computer and remove corrupt information held within the cell memory. This reformatting sets the stage for the communication of the correct information shared by all of the cells within the body by allowing the true information to flow into these freshly "rebooted" or "flashed" memory mediums (David Stewart, 2009).

Foods Measured on the ORAC Scale

There have been recent scientific breakthroughs in the form of two different "tools" meant for measurement purposes. The first is a laboratory procedure used to calculate the antioxidant capabilities of a food. ORAC, or oxygen radical absorption capability, is a scale that has been created to represent this. Berries, greens, and legumes in comparison to other types of foods have the highest rating on the ORAC scale, with wolfberries being the highest. Of course these measurements were taken with the foods in their most pristine condition, alive and vibrant.

Wolfberries are the highest rated food on the ORAC scale with a rating of 25,300 (umTE/100gm). Always be sure when you look at a foods ORAC rating that the comparisons of different food items being tested have used the same units of measurement. If these berries and greens are so powerful and are full of this absorption capability, what about the capabilities of these essential oils? After all, these oils are *concentrated* versions of these plants and should have higher ORAC readings.

Essential oils tip the scales with scores topping these berries. The reason for this is due to its concentrated characteristics. We said wolfberries had a rating of 25,300 (umTE/100gm), whereas clove oil has a rating of 1,078,700 (umTE/100gm). What this tells us is that essential oils can be the best forms of antioxidants found on earth, offering the most free radical neutralization available, which provides the most effective anti-aging, cleansing, and alkalizing properties (David Stewart, 2009).

The Measurement of Nano-Frequencies

Another new tool is a sensitive frequency analyzer developed by Bruce Tainio of Tainio Industries in Cheny, Washington. This tool was created to measure nano-frequencies. Nano (one billionth) frequencies are too faint to pick up and measure with conventional frequency analyzing equipment. Frequencies are a direct representation of electrical activity, in the case of a plant or animal, a representation of life force.

Fresh herbs have a frequency of 20–27 MHz, dried herbs 12-22 MHz. Fresh produce measured 5-10 MHz, canned and processed food measured zero (not absolute zero, as even inanimate objects have a frequency) as its life force has been rendered kaput. The reason for lack of electrical activity is due to the lack of life force within. This tells us that processed foods are dead and therefore can never provide life-sustaining nutrients.

A healthy individual will have a reading from 62-68 MHz, with lower frequencies when we are sick. Below 58 MHz can lead to colds, 57MHz is where the flu will manifest itself. Candida yeast infestations occur at 55 MHz and Epstein-Barr syndrome at 52 MHz. Cancer begins when the cells fall below 42 MHz, and death starts at 25 MHz and ends at zero (David Stewart, 2009).

Free Radicals at It Again

Free radicals, or positively charged ions, can interrupt electrical activity; as a result, they lower a body's frequencies. We should see, based on the different stages from being healthy with a high frequency, to zero at death. We want to maintain a higher frequency within the body. This is because frequency is a direct representation of the electrical activity, and high-electrical activity in the body tells us that the body's systems are communicating with one another and functioning properly.

Essential Oils Win Again

Essential oils carry higher frequencies that, when used by other living things, will facilitate the heightening of that body's frequency. The lowest frequency oil is still higher than any fresh herb or vegetable, from the lowest frequency being from the oil of basil at 52 MHz, to the highest reading from the oil of rose at 320 MHz. Because these frequencies are so high, they have the ability to raise our frequencies to a level where illness and disease cannot manifest or survive. Einstein knew that when you mix two different frequencies, you end up with one new frequency. When you use high-frequency essential oils, it raises your frequency!

As I said, you need to add alkaline elements to your body's solution for pH balance, so when you do so, you want to add heavily concentrated forms of alkaline sources (natural) to your body's internal environment. The more alkali you add, the more effective it will be at raising your pH. At the same time, if you want to increase the overall frequency that your body emits, it makes sense that by exposing ourselves to high-frequency oils, you achieve higher or concentrated frequencies within the body as well. Just like chemistry, when you mix two chemicals together that will react on a molecular level, the resulting chemical is different from the original (chemical reaction). At the same time, when you mix two frequencies, the resulting frequency is different from the original two.

It was also found that these frequencies can be affected in different ways by the (hora) frequency of the surrounding life forces (this concept was proven by Edison and Einstein). Einstein said that the brain is a transmitter and receiver of frequency and that these frequencies are really energy in the form of vibration, similar to radio waves. It was also proven that these vibrations that are being emitted by the brain can affect the surrounding matter.

It has also been proven scientifically that a positive frequency (thought) is hundreds of times more powerful than a negative one. Later it was shown that a negative attitude or negative thoughts can actually *lower* the frequencies of these essential oils. At the same time, if the oils are placed in the vicinity of positive, happy people, these frequencies were *raised*.

Spiritual Connection with Healing Oils

This tells us that prayer (intent) and spiritual connection are imperative to gain the full health benefits of these oils. They respond to our needs by asking of them what it is that we want from them, thus responding to us in a favorable manner. Moses said that God will bless the oils of a righteous person (Exodus 28:41, 29:7, 29:36, 30:26, 30:30, 40:9, 40:10, 40:11, 40:13, 40:14). Measuring the frequency of an essential oil that has been blessed is scientific proof that this is true. Oils can work without prayer and prayer can work without oils, but when you use the two in conjunction, they become exponentially more powerful. The two techniques used together takes into consideration addressing chemical contamination as well as spiritual or electrical chaos (spiritual for me means simply electrical or having to do with energy) within the body.

Unnatural Foods Never Work

Food items that have been ruined through production and processing (among other things) have the ability to lower your body's frequencies. Changing things from their natural state in different ways causes the creation of free radicals, including simply overcooking them or even cooking them at all.

Just holding a cup of coffee can reduce your frequency by 8 MHz; taking a sip can lower it by 14 MHz. This is a perfect example of how processing destroys the healing properties of a food, as coffee is one of the top ten types of antioxidant foods (along with dark chocolate) in its pristine condition. After it has been roasted and processed, it loses this anti-aging, antioxidant property. If you're already slightly low in frequency, consuming your everyday coffee product can lower your body's frequency enough to put you in ranges where illness can begin. Any food item overly processed and dead will cause this undesired effect (David Stewart, 2009).

I talked about mixing these oils together to get even better results in healing. These mixes (elixirs) are often referred to as *blends*. As there are many different types of oils, there can be even more different types of blends. Joy, Valor, Exodus II, Thieves, three Wise Men—to name a few blends available—originated up to thousands of years ago and are still available today! The names of these blends being used today are not necessarily the original names given to them by their creators, as they are ancient and were passed on by recipe through hundreds of years. Some of these names are trademarks of essential oil producers.

Formula Handed Down by God

Exodus II is the name of a blend that was originally created by Moses in the book of Exodus. This formula was handed down to him directly from the Almighty himself (through spiritual connection with God, inspired thought). This formula consists of olive oil (carrier), cassia, myrrh, cinnamon, calamus, hyssop, galbanum, frankincense, and spikenard. This blend was to be the holy anointing oil, as it has healing, spiritual energy, and meditative capabilities and was used in synagogues and churches for centuries.

I have a friend who is a Hindu, and he has *sacred* oils that he receives and gives blessings with, again reinforcing that this was not meant so much to be a proprietary ritual to any specific religious denomination, but that this was meant to be done by all people to help facilitate optimum health. People from different cultures and different religious backgrounds used a lot of the same oils for their holy anointments of one another. This was due to the fact that these oils came from the same regions or through trade routes in these areas.

Special Blends Used for Centuries

Valor is a blend used by the Spartans and the Romans, among other soldiers throughout history, during training, before battle, and during movements. This oil is used to give the person courage and strength. The healing characteristics of this blend contain oils with the same frequencies as bones and joints, which help line up the spine and facilitate the healing of skeletal deficiencies. This blend consists of spruce, rosewood, blue tansy, frankincense, and almond oil (David Stewart, 2009).

Joy is an exotic blend of essential oils that creates magnetic energy within the body. This helps create a sensation of bliss. This blend is often used to stimulate romance between lovers or create a feeling of togetherness among family and friends. Ingredients are bergamot, ylang-ylang, geranium, rosewood, lemon, mandarin, jasmine, Roman chamomile, palmarosa, and rose (David Stewart, 2009).

Thieves is a special blend of oils used by some savvy alchemists during the time of the Great Plague in France during the renaissance. This blend allowed criminals to enter the homes of the dead and steal their goods without contracting the plague. They were able to come and go *before* the dead were removed by the authorities. Often times the bodies were left behind, as the authorities were too afraid of contracting the plague themselves, yet these thieves came and went unscathed (David Stewart, 2009).

The authorities managed to capture some of these thieves and demanded an explanation as to how they pulled it off. By offering a lesser sentence, these people found out from the thieves that it was a special blend of essential oils that had been used to ward off the disease. Thieves is still available today and is an excellent tool for fighting microbial infestation (cold, flu) and for supporting the immune system. There are all kinds of cleaning products made with this special blend for your home today. Thieves has also been used successfully to shorten the duration of a cold sore to about three days by a personal friend. This person used to take Valtrex every day to prevent the onset of cold sores, as they had been so severe and frequent in the past. After she began her clean regime, she discontinued the use of the drug since she got a cold sore anyway while taking it, and because Thieves worked so well at getting rid of it. She thought the cost and possible side effects weren't worth the risk in taking Valtrex every day. Thieves blend consists of clove, lemon, cinnamon, eucalyptus, and rosemary (David Stewart, 2009).

Another blend that I like to use is Three Wise Men. I'm sure most of us have heard of the three wise men, as they were the three kings that brought gifts to Mary, Joseph, and baby Jesus in Bethlehem on his birthday. And what were two out of these three gifts? They were essential oils. Surely these oils must have been considered valuable and sacred, considering these were the gifts that kings brought for the Son of God on the night of his birth. Needless to say, these oils were very valuable and held sacred by the people of this time because they understood the health benefits of these oils. Ingredients: sandalwood, juniper, frankincense, spruce, and myrrh in a carrier of almond oil (David Stewart, 2009).

Purity Is Always Important

Like any other plant-based therapeutic compound, essential oils need to be derived from clean, organically grown, toxin-free vegetation in order to have a positive cleansing ability and overall detoxifying effect on the body. Using oils made from contaminated vegetation can be exponentially more dangerous than eating contaminated vegetables or produce. Because oils are concentrated from large amounts of vegetation (150 lbs of leaves might equal a quart of oil), if the plants, leaves, woods, or barks are loaded with unnatural chemicals, these toxins will become concentrated as well.

This is also dangerous because the foreign substances can react with the favorable compounds within the oils and turn them into other potentially dangerous or toxic compounds. So be sure you choose oils that come from vegetation that was organically or responsibly grown and derived by a reliable company or person who understands how to produce truly therapeutic essential oils. Most oils that are sold at retailers are manmade and not to be used therapeutically, if at all.

A Message from the Creator

"And thou shalt make it an oil of holy ointment, an ointment compound after the art of the apothecary: it shall be an holy anointing oil." Exodus 30:25, "And the anointing oil, and sweet incense for the holy place: according to all that I have commanded thee shall they do" (Exodus 31:11. 25:6, 29:7, 29:21, 30:31, 31:11, 35:8, 35:15, 35:28). Like I've said before, everything we *need* has been given to us by the Creator. Essential oils have been used by all faiths and cultures throughout history.

Aromatherapy also consists of burning incense. This is another way to release the therapeutic oils from the herbs, wood, bark, or leaves. God instructed Moses to burn or heat leaves and barks as well as use oils. People have used these techniques for thousands of years. Smoking is a form of aromatherapy, but like anything else, it needs to be done in an informed and intelligent manner. American Indians smoked tobacco but did not suffer from debilitating disease as a result.

All Cultures throughout Ancient History

Oils and incense were used on a daily basis by people in the past; it was commonplace in the household and lifestyle. Oils were shared, traded, and looked upon as treasured gifts. People in the ancient past might not have understood the science in the way we do today, but they *knew* that they were to be used and why they should be used: to achieve and maintain optimum health. They had faith in the use of the tools that God the Creator left behind for them. This concept has been lost and suppressed for too long and needs to be looked at in a productive and intelligent manner, so essential oils can be reintroduced as tools of healthy living for all people of all faiths once again.

Dangers of Supplements

There are so many different supplements out there from your average daily vitamins to complete body detoxification programs. It's hard to know what to choose or if you should use any of them at all! Most of these supplements claiming to have all-natural ingredients and are safe to use as a result. There are, however, a few reasons why these supplements, although sometimes consisting of natural substances, can still pose health risks.

Drug Companies at It Again

Drug companies try to change laws requiring prescriptions for the acquisition of vitamins. Needless to say this hasn't happened yet (thank God), as this would most likely be detrimental to our freedom to obtain natural substances as well as having costs greatly increased. But it is the same reason that companies with less integrity (greed) can offer you an all-natural product that really isn't.

Food companies are only required to have actually equal to or greater than 70 percent all-natural components within their product in order to carry the label all-natural of said foods per regulations of the FDA. The FDA also stated that the term *natural* shall remain undefined in the food and cosmetic industries. The companies that are stating an actual number representing a percentage of all-natural ingredients are more honest or accurate in the description of the content of their food product. If a product is truly all natural, then it should state 100 percent natural. If it says all natural, it is probably closer to 70 percent natural, which leaves a lot of room for unnatural ingredients. If a product is really high in natural content then the company selling it should want to brag about the actual percentage of natural ingredients by advertising the actual percentage of natural ingredients included in the recipe.

Again, if it is truly all natural, it should say 100 percent natural. All natural does not mean 100 percent natural. Keep in mind that even 100 percent natural products may still have been exposed to unnatural chemicals during its procurement. Again, these substances, since not put there as part of the recipe, do not have to be mentioned in the ingredients; only certified organic food products are actually 100 percent natural. This is true whether the components were intended in the ingredients or not.

Jumping on the Bandwagon

Companies are jumping on the bandwagon due to the major shift taking place in the minds of people around the world considering natural and organic foods as healthier choices. As a result there are many products carrying the label "all natural" that are very close to this accusation and are very safe to consume. At the same time, there are many other products that aren't safe, yet are carrying the label "healthy," all the while these products contain many dangerous artificial substances despite the efforts to convince you otherwise.

Oftentimes when companies focus on a familiar term like HFCS, stating on the label how it isn't among the ingredients, it is often a distraction from the fact that there are other dangerous chemicals not identified on the label, at least not in big letters on the front. Sometimes when we see a label that says "no artificial flavors" we think it is healthy, but the fact is that this is only one of many chemicals being used by food producers.

Know the Source

The same is true for supplements; the best way to know if these products are what they should be is to grow and create them yourself. In most cases this is nearly impossible if you want to take advantage of all the herbal vegetation out there. The next best way would be to know the sources of the supplements you want to take. For example, if you want to know if your organic, whole-food antioxidant supplement is actually that, you could go to the factory and farms to see for yourself that this is true.

This isn't a bad idea but for the most part would be difficult to accomplish. This could be another reason why buying local can be beneficial. Granted, this is an extreme idea, especially since most of us do absolutely nothing to see that we are buying and consuming safe food and supplement products. This is mostly because we trust the *big* companies that show happy, healthy people on TV using their products. We all fall for these marketing deceptions whether we realize it or not.

This is why there was the idea for a predetermined set of rules to be used as a standard of quality and purity of food cultivation and production. This is done by a third party and certified as so. This certification process is called "certified organic." Organics are the best way for us to know that what we are exposing ourselves to is safe. Realize that, in the business world, there exists greed and corruption that always leaves the possibility for deception, but if you consume organic food on a regular basis, you'll learn that there are major differences in taste and quality. So even if you are a skeptic for the certification process, because you're thinking there is room for corruption in this area as well (and there is), the consistent use of organic products will teach you the difference for yourself. Many people like myself (friends) who have made the switch to organics for an extended period of time cannot eat everyday, regular food like they used to because it makes them sick and just doesn't taste as good.

Taking Apart Nature's Formulas

Next to carrying the organic certification, the next characteristic goes hand in hand with the first as it is just as important. All supplements, food choices, etc., need to be chosen for their whole-food status. "Whole food" means that we are consuming foods as they exist in nature, with all its parts intact. Nature has already put together the *proper* formulas and should not be altered. A bad habit of chemists and manufacturers, even in the truly natural group, is to find a natural food with healing properties, try to figure which of the many compounds within the plant are beneficial, and then extracting them and sell it isolated from the other components within the natural "formulas."

Exposure to Isolated Compounds

Exposure to these isolated compounds can be detrimental to our health. When we consume certain vitamins and compounds isolated from food sources, we can cause a chemical imbalance within the body. Cofactors exist between different types of vitamins, minerals, enzymes, where the consumption of an isolated compound found in natural food can deplete other elements or compounds found naturally within the body. An example of this would be taking zinc if you think you're getting a cold to boost your immune system, the problem is that too much zinc will deplete your copper stores.

Are Everyday Vitamins Safe?

Conventional vitamin complexes such as Ultra Megas and Theras are vitamin supplements that do not conform to this all-natural, whole-food concept. These vitamin and supplement companies try to put together a formula that is as good or even superior to nature's formulas. This colored, hard pill made of what seems to be rocks and extracts is far from a whole-food supplement.

The average vitamins on the market today should not be considered healthy or consumed at all. Unless of course if you were stuck on a deserted island with no food source other than the most popular fast food restaurant, along with a steady supply of mainstream vitamins available to you, then taking these vitamins with your meals would be beneficial. If you do take these kinds of vitamins, you should always take them with a well-balanced meal. Ironically, if you do eat healthy, high-quality, well-balanced meals, you won't need to take vitamins.

We Can Make Better Choices

Most of us are not stuck on a deserted or isolated island forced to eat nothing but fast food (with vitamins); therefore, we have the ability to eat healthier food and find healthier supplements. Supplements are a good way to supplement the nutrients that you don't get from your diet. It is always better, however, to eat a complete diet consisting of many different organic vegetables, including heavy greens, quality organic and wild meats, organic whole grains, and fresh organic produce. This will ensure you're getting the nutrition you need without supplements. However, supplements are a valuable resource to have on hand for occasional use, again when you have lapses within your diet plan or even on semi-regular use.

How Many Supplements to Use

There may be some supplements you want to use on a regular basis, but these are limited, again, if you're eating a balanced, nutrient-rich diet of quality foods. One such supplement for regular use is the mineral supplement added to make the optimum healthy water for hydration, for two reasons. First adding minerals to your diet is a very good idea, and second because it provides you with the optimum water source for hydration.

Another good supplement to use a few times a week is organic, raw apple cider vinegar (unfiltered). This can be used to cure acid reflux disease as well as help maintain proper pH in the body. This is an example of an acid that has an alkalizing effect on the body. This can be used every day if you want, as you would any vinegar.

Natural Medicines and Natural Supplements

There are all-natural medicines out there sold as remedies for cold symptoms, infections, and other ailments. These are better alternatives to artificial compounds as remedies but still do not always follow the concept of whole food and should not be considered whole-food supplements. Many are safe to use as remedies on a short-term basis but should never be used long term.

Any health problems should be addressed by a licensed healthcare professional. Seeing a nutritionist or an ND can help solve nutritional deficiencies and help you decide which food and or whole-food supplement products to use. You will want to make sure they stay true to the concept of all natural whole-food supplements as well as food and cosmetics.

Whole Food Concept Reinforced

So we want to make sure that our supplements are made from whole foods, herbs, plants, and other foods. *Truly* all natural is always the best and safest way to go. Here is a list of supplements that I use:

Organic, Pure Super-Smoothie Recipe

(All in powdered form used in morning smoothie)

- Organic green complex

- Alkaline mineral complex

- Fiber supplement

- Psyllium fiber

- Structuring, alkalizing, ionic water additives used in distilled water as drinking and cooking water

- Organic antioxidant complex (capsule form taken twice a week)

Smoothie recipe:

2 organic whole eggs

1 heaping tsp. greens

1 tsp. both fibers

1 tsp. alkaline minerals

16 oz. healthy water

2 tbsp. pure honey

1 whole banana

1/4 c. organic rolled oats

In a blender, combine water, banana, honey, and egg whites. Measure out oatmeal in a cup; add fibers, greens, and minerals. Blend original mixture on high for ten seconds. Add oatmeal mixture and blend on high thoroughly. If you are too scared to eat raw eggs or if eggs are not part of your diet for whatever reason, they can be omitted and replaced with another protein source. I have been eating this breakfast for many years now.

Unless I have an ailment, I do not use any other supplements on a regular basis. As far as drug use, I do not use any, not even aspirin. I try to maintain a consistent amount of fresh vegetation in my diet. This has kept me feeling young and vibrant for years now, and I believe this will continue to be true for years to come.

Always consult a licensed healthcare professional to help you make better choices in nutrition. No one has all the definitive answers to all the mysteries of the world, including food, health, chemistry, and physics. Every day we find out something new that we didn't know a day earlier; sometimes findings are the addition of beneficial natural concepts, other times we find out that what we *have* been doing for years to stay healthy is actually unhealthy.

Corporations and Politics

Healthcare a For-Profit Business

It is an atrocity that the healthcare industry was ever created as a for-profit business. They try to con you with the idea that we have state-of-the-art healthcare, specialists, and companies providing technologies and medicines that far outpace the healthcare of the rest of the world and that other countries which offer "free" healthcare cannot compete and heal the way we do.

This concept is a lie perpetuated by the corporate machine that is the United States healthcare system. Last time I checked, we ranked thirty-seventh in the world for healing and being healthy as a country (Librarian50, 2012). It doesn't sound like the trillions of dollars that are being spent and earned every year are actually helping us become healthier. Yet we continue to buy into the belief that we have the greatest healthcare system and the best medicines in the world.

Our Western Ancestors Would Never Take It

Oddly enough, some other countries would never put up with the healthcare system that we have in this country. It is our silence and apathy that led to our ridiculously huge and corrupt healthcare system. Not that their systems are perfect; I'm sure they're all going broke at the same time from the corporate and political greed throwing their weight around in their world as well. Losing your health has become another means for the corporate machine to fleece you of your hard-earned money.

Is There Superior Medicine in the USA?

We do not have superior medicine in this country, as we spend too much time and money trying to reinvent nature, addressing only symptomatic problems and not addressing the real causes of afflictions. Healthcare has become such a high-profit business that it has become an imperative part of the economy and would hurt too many businesses if corruption were to be eliminated in the healthcare industry. Eliminating corruption by actually providing affordable cures and healing for people, setting them free from any financial burdens they would normally endure along with their ailments, would devastate the healthcare industry.

By affordable I mean affordable to everyone, even the poor who have very little money, because everyone deserves affordable healthcare. I'm not talking about the out-of-touch politicians and very rich peoples' idea of what is affordable. At this point I don't think they even know what that is. Some of these people are so used to looking at gigantic piles of money they are out of touch with the financial realities of the average person today. Even though they know *you* are broke, they still can't relate to being so themselves.

Quality Surgeons and
Drugs Have to Be Expensive

US drugs and surgeries that use new techniques and inventions are expensive because they have to be, right? I mean, that's what makes them superior to the others, correct? Reality again is that this is a façade perpetuated through the TV, brainwashing us into believing that this is true. And with so many people sick and nowhere else to turn, it seems like the only hope for us when we are sick, is running to the doctors to get all of the drugs and surgeries that are constantly advertised on television.

Drug Companies Importing Active Ingredients

Drug companies often import their active ingredients from other poorer or less-developed countries as they are available at a much lower cost, further maximizing profits for the company. According to a US-Niagara Trading Corp's advertisement, they specialize in importing active pharmaceutical ingredients that are used in many everyday drugs from overseas for distribution in the U.S. (US Niagara Trading Corp, 2012). *Wait!* Importing active ingredients from other less-developed, poorer countries? If that is the case, doesn't that mean essentially I am not doing business with a high-tech, superior American company in the end anyway? Just like everything else, these things are probably all made out of the country, as we manufacture much less these days, due to the increasing costs of living and doing business here.

Personally it has become very difficult for me to actually make any money in the construction business, because the costs of goods and doing business are too high in relation to what people can afford to pay and what things used to cost only a few years ago. In order to get jobs, I have to bid them lower than I was in 2000, yet the cost of gas, materials, insurances, and everything else has gone up exponentially. I found this hard to believe until I sat down and looked at my old financial reports.

Downside of Publicly Traded Corporations

The problem with a publicly traded company is that shareholders can be directly involved with basic business operations and hold positions within the company; at the same time, they can be an investor but have no part of the general operations of the company. It leaves the people who do run the company legally bound to do whatever it takes to make the other uninvolved investors as much money as possible.

So if a public business venture is not profitable, it will be sold, liquidated, or it will collapse while the shareholders move on to another business they can invest in. Someone like I have no choice but to "keep on keeping on," as this is the only way I earn a living. I don't have the ability to just raise my prices at will to satisfy my financial needs and goals. Instead I have to work harder, longer, and even create other sources of income, which takes up more free time.

This is exactly what goes on in politics and in big businesses that control the world's provisions. For as long as we have lived in a society, this has been true and continues to be so. Again, there is nothing wrong with free enterprise and the earning of a comfortable living as long as you consider if you are hurting others or not. It only makes sense that the healthier and richer your customers are, the healthier and richer you will be. Healthy people and healthy society (honor, integrity, care for others) equals healthy economy for all.

Business Ethics: an Oath to Live By

I fully realize that no wealth or position can long endure, unless built upon truth and justice; therefore, I will enter into no transaction that does not benefit all who it affects. I will succeed by attracting to myself the forces I wish to use and the cooperation of other people. I will induce others to serve me because of my willingness to serve others. I will eliminate hatred, envy, jealousy, selfishness, and cynicism by developing love for all humanity, because I know a negative attitude toward others can never bring me success. I will cause others to believe in me, because I will believe in them and myself.

(Napoleon Hill, Think and Grow Rich, 2009).

Washington, Business, Politics, and Lobbyists

This is not all business, but the larger corrupt corporations that have the ability to manipulate the system with their lobbyist-politician relationships, as well as simply having enough money to do so, are the ones you need to watch out for. The idea of a corporation itself is not an evil thing, and further I believe it can be done in a productive, sustainable manner (which is happening every day), where all involved with the business are well taken care of, as long as they do a good job and the business profits, with a good wage and recognition for their efforts.

It sickens me to think of large groups of people being taken advantage of by small groups of bloodsucking elite that know other people are desperate, offering salaries that barely allow them to maintain a living at all. Never mind the quality of life that they deserve as hardworking, productive people. But they know that the common man needs a job and will eventually do whatever he has to in order to provide for his or her family. As a result, these companies make record profits and don't want to share this with the people who actually helped make the money in the first place.

Enough for Everyone to Live Well and Prosper

Everyone involved (employees, officers, investors) with any
company is an integral part of its day-to-day operations,
production, and resulting profit. There are some private
corporations with people who believe in and have implemented
this concept where everyone involved with the creation of profit
get paid accordingly with good wages (wages one can live and
prosper on) and profit sharing (Michael Moore, 2009). As a result,
production, morale, and lifestyle have been completely turned
around, as they are happy to go to work every day and are able to
prosper at the same time. This is possible because everyone who
profits from this company is *directly* involved with its operation,
and the profits are evenly shared.

More Problems with the Public Corporation

Another problem with the average publicly traded company is
that there are typically too many people trying to take too much
profit from a business without doing anything at all to operate,
run, improve, or help production in any way. Ironically, in the
end, the investors are the people who are *prioritized* above the
consumers (fellow citizens) and especially the actual workers
who toil on a daily basis to make it all happen in the first place.
This is a problem for me, not because I'm envious or even care
about other people's greedy ambitions or financial windfalls, but
because I can see the damage it is doing to the country, economy,
environment, and, more importantly, people's lives.

Corporations Are an Integral Part of Society

Publicly traded corporations can be an integral part of a society's development in many ways. It took large amounts of money to create such huge organized developments in manufacturing and industry, which lead to a never-ending source of materials for application of new technologies. The problem is once again greed. I realize if the money wasn't available, then these types of ventures would not be possible; however, ambitious, hardworking, simple people who work their entire lives devoted to a company should be rewarded for their hard work as well.

At the same time these things would not be possible if it were not for all of the people involved, making each employee an integral part of making it all happen. Just because someone has more money than another doesn't make the richer person more important than the poorer. Nor is the person who happened to come up with a good idea for something profitable; because if they hadn't, someone else would have sooner or later, and most likely they would not have been able to make their idea a reality by themselves.

I have all kinds of big ideas coming to mind every day, but without the help of other people, I cannot make them a reality myself. Let's face it, even as an author with the ability to write a book alone, you still cannot have success without other people. So as an investor you should be no more important to the possibilities of profit and therefore should not make upward of 90 percent plus of all the monies being created from the people working toward those profits.

A New Policing Governmental Agency

We have learned the hard way that we cannot trust big business. This is why we have so many new policing-type administrations being created to monitor the actions of all these different areas of industry and commerce. So, it would make sense to trust in the government to protect you, right? Well, it would be nice, but the problem is that the government is all about business and nothing more. They make it look like they are working for you when in reality they are working for the guy with a financial interest in whatever their administration is policing and themselves, of course. The government is so big now that it has become a special interest group itself.

I need you to realize that I do not believe in one gigantic, organized governmental conspiracy, as I believe it is an impossible and a ridiculous concept. The government is too big, and there is no way to have everyone involved in one large conspiracy collectively. However, there is plenty of room for special interest groups to use their money and power to manipulate the laws and government to act in their favor. Unfortunately, this is how things are done today through the use of lobbyists, partnerships, payoffs, campaign contributions, extortion, and conspiracy, which is really only scratching the surface as to how these groups go about changing things to their favor.

Does the FDA Effectively Protect You?

How does the FDA really know what a pharmaceutical company is selling? They would have to be chemists and actually take place in the research and development of these chemicals themselves in order to know if products are safe for exposure to humans. This must be true, as these are the people who protect us from dangerous food, drugs, and cosmetics.

The reality is they can't and don't know what these compounds do except for what the manufacturer presents to them. They basically have a specific guideline for procedures in order to create, test, and manufacture new drugs. These procedures are laws that can be changed by the pharmaceutical companies with their lobbyists, giving them the ability to make their own rules for these procedures, which is what they've done. This is why new drugs today get approved by the FDA, only to find out six to twelve months later that thousands of people have died from it, and a few hundred thousand people have had adverse side effects, and now there is a class-action lawsuit against the company that made the drug. Funny, no matter how many lawsuits they have against them due to bad drugs they make, they still manage to stay in business.

Does Your Doctor Know What He Is Prescribing?

How about your doctor? I'm pretty sure he is not a chemist. Yes, he probably took some 1000–2000 level chemistry courses in order to get his degree, but he most likely doesn't know squat about these chemicals that he is prescribing, except of course for what the manufacturer of the drug told him about it through advertising, articles in medical publishing, and clinical studies. And yet this technique is predominantly what is being done to remedy our afflictions today! Like the FDA, the doctors just go with whatever the drug companies say about it because the FDA said they verify it.

This idea really started to bother me because I had to throw away my naïve and trusting way of thinking and be a little more skeptical when it comes to the realities of big business. So the question comes down to: whom can you trust? The answer is simple really. We need to re-learn how to put our trust in God the Creator. You don't need to be religious to love, respect, and know that you come from the earth and are directly connected to the earth, as well as one another. The reality is that everything we need to stay happy and healthy—physically, spiritually, mentally, and emotionally—is already here on earth, given to us by the Creator.

If this is true, then why do we always try to reinvent the wheel and come up with new foods, medicines, and hygiene products? The reason is greed once again. Unfortunately, there are people out there who care more about money than other people.

I Believe in Free Enterprise without Pain

I don't want to sound like I'm against free enterprise, because I am definitely not. I am a business owner, and I am grateful to our forefathers and all the soldiers who have provided me with the freedom to own and operate my own business. However, I believe that doing business in this country, or anywhere for that matter, should be recognized as a privilege and should not be allowed if the business does not contribute to the greater good of the people involved with providing that same business's wealth. That means employees as well as customers. In other words, I don't think anyone has the right to free enterprise when it hurts or does damage to people or the planet.

Yes, obviously this concept of doing business correctly with ethics and integrity is nothing new. We have Ivy League business schools teaching about business ethics; we have all kinds of government in place to police these businesses, right? Despite all the efforts, it seems plenty of things are being done the wrong way, and the answer to why again is greed perpetuated by the bloodsucking elite all the way down to the average individual.

Health insurance costs went up 32 percent this year in the state of Massachusetts (my brother is sixty-three this year and pays $1,500-plus a month for he and his wife to be covered with health insurance). These facts make it even more difficult for people and small businesses to hire, as the costs are too great as it is, and the economy is so weak that we are all working for and making less money! However, politicians (and their friends) just seem to keep making more every day. But what happens when the money runs out? Don't our leaders think about the future of this country?

Massachusetts business owners hoped to get relief this year from the overburdening costs of health insurance, for the restoration of prosperity to local business (small) increasing their ability to hire and profit. As usual the decisions were made to benefit the larger, more powerful, and corrupt corporations. The regulatory administration and the governor have stated repeatedly that they are doing everything they can to increase jobs by keeping the costs of health insurance and other operating expenses down (other insurance and taxes), as healthcare is such an overwhelming expense for small business as it is.

With the inevitable increase of these costs, it's painfully obvious to see who these people work for. Yes, the politicians have sold us out; it doesn't matter what their name is, what party they claim membership, or who their friends are. They and their friends (corporations, lobbyists) have an agenda as usual, and it does not include the public or consumers, only themselves and their friends. This type of practice is commonplace in government today and does not provide for a sustainable economy. Without jobs there is no income; without income there is no spending (among many other tragic happenstances); without spending there is no economy and the eventual collapse of society!

We need to community-up and take care of ourselves again as our forefathers and ancestors did. We might not like the idea; it sounds scary and uncomfortable, but I think that soon we won't have a choice. We need to be self-reliant and sufficient, grow food, conserve resources, recycle, tend to the environment, create our own clean energy, and so on, as a citizenry together, without the need to let others do it for us (politicians and corporations). However, without education and health, it will be a near impossibility, so join me in getting back to the basics so we can move more swiftly into the future of harmony and technology within society and economics.

The stage is set for this to happen. As more of us lose our jobs, we will be looking for a way to sustain life for ourselves and our families. These concepts may be the only choice we will have. With major changes happening in the economy and technology (through necessity and mistakes), there will be more opportunities for people to start small local business, again, pertaining to some of the basics like food and energy. It takes a healthy, productive, creative mind to build the future.

Stress and Energetic Rebalancing

Stress is something we are all aware of today with the failing economy, wars, natural disasters, financial woes, illness, and many other sources. However, when we get stressed we need to relax. I don't think we realize just how damaging stress can be to our overall health.

Different Types of Stresses

There are two types of stress we experience; one is the physical kind, which happens when our bodies are overworked and fatigued. This happens often to us today, as we have very busy schedules, and it is very hard to earn a living for most people right now. Many have to work multiple jobs just to make ends meet and do not get nearly enough sleep. Others, by the time they do make it to bed, can't sleep anyway due to not the physical stress but the other kind of stress that we experience more and more today.

Another form of physical stress is placed in the body when it is overwhelmed with contamination. This is another form of physical stress and leaves the body subject to dysfunction, breakdown, and injury. Unlike the other form of physical stress, this type of stress can happen without us realizing it. It takes place within the body without us knowing it. Oftentimes we think when we sustain a physical injury, that it should have happened or it would have happened to any healthy person under those circumstances. Sometimes this is true, but oftentimes we sustain injury due to existing physical stress, which is hidden from the obvious, until we fall down or bump our elbow and sustain a serious injury.

Why is it that children bounce back a lot quicker and easier from what seem like serious falls? Ironically it's true that children do seem to handle some serious falls as miraculous saves, but at the same time children are a lot more fragile and susceptible to injury from internal physical stress (chemical and microbial contamination).

Mental Stress: the Big Problem

Mental stress is a much bigger problem. A good night's rest is not necessarily the answer and may be impossible, especially if your stresses are causing insomnia. Mental stress can lead not only to more physical stress through sleep deprivation but can cause all kinds of health problems as well. Mental stresses (emotional traumas) are not stored within the brain's memory center. These types of memories are stored within the memory of our cells throughout the body.

When we experience these traumatic events, they can be stored anywhere in the body that can later manifest themselves with physical illness (dysfunction). This is one of the reasons that stress can be so dangerous if it is not dealt with correctly. Also, mental stress can seriously degrade the body and the brain, resulting in dysfunction of the body's systems.

Manage Current and Future Stresses

Just like chemical contamination, we want to eliminate not only current and future sources of contamination but also deal with previous contaminants that are currently stored in the body as well. The same is true for these stresses. They need to be dealt with on two levels; one is to find a way to manage and eliminate existing stresses that are either causing problems now or could pop up in the future. Second is to deal with stored painful stresses, emotions, or traumas from the past that are stored away in our bodies and need to be dealt with and put to rest.

Physical stress is, most of the time, easily fixed with rest and proper nutrition for our bodies. But mental stress isn't as easily remedied because it can be a powerful force and have many different causes. The obvious triggers would be troubles that we may be having with money, health problems of loved ones, our health, relationships, and so forth. These stresses can exist within our bodies as they are left behind from past bad experiences and emotional traumas. There might be triggers that we are aware of that remind us of prior bad experiences, but we can have these things manifest themselves from causes that we are unaware of as well.

Stress Can Impede the Immune System

Stress can lower the immune system by throwing the body electrically or spiritually out of balance. This can cause dysfunction within the body, leading to all kinds of illnesses, including irritability, nervous breakdowns, panic attacks, psychosis, depression, and many other physical and mental health problems. We should also realize that stress creates a lot of acid within the body, which as we have learned can cause a lowering of the overall pH of the body's intra-cellular fluids. When this happens, it sets us up for any type of disorder or dysfunction within the body. Besides stress affecting our electrical systems, there are also other sources of interference of these systems that come in the form of magnetic fields (EMF).

Energetic Rebalancing Forms of Therapy

Energetic rebalancing is a generalized term describing the different therapies or techniques used in the rebalancing of our electrical system. Along with cleaning our bodies of contaminants, we may also need to get our wiring back in order. This is how we address the existing problems that are affecting us right now, from things in the past, stress, and EMF sources. The next thing we will do is to take a look at dealing with the current and future sources of these EMFs by way of shielding. "Shielding" is a term describing the means of protecting one frequency from another, so the weaker frequency is not interrupted by the stronger one.

Shielding Techniques for the Body

Shielding the body is accomplished a few basic ways; one is by using magnets, either wearing them as jewelry or using seat cushions and bedding with magnets in them. Magnets are used to shield all kinds of devices from exterior EMFs, such as the cable of your computer monitor. If you've ever noticed the "line wart" or cylindrical-looking object that wraps the wire near the source, that's a magnet. I have a bracelet that has magnets in it to help shield myself from EMFs.

Maybe you have seen a "magical bracelet" that does wonderful things to improve health and overall performance. This technology has everything to do with these shielding concepts that we are talking about. By shielding our bodies, we are better protecting ourselves from these dangerous EMFs, which allow our body's electrical system and all subsequent systems thereafter to function more properly.

Implosion Technology Used for Shielding

Another form of shielding is accomplished through the use of implosion technology. This is water that is magnetized in such a way that it acts as an EMF shield. This water can be held in all types and sizes of containing devices and then is used as a shield from many household and office sources of these EMFs. These come made for TVs and monitors, as these are continuous sources of strong EMFs in our environment.

Essential Oils at It Again

Essential oils not only protect and cleanse the body of chemical contamination, but they can also protect the body from harmful effects of EMFs. Essential oils can protect us from all kinds of electrical bombardment including X-rays, radiations, microwaves, etc.

We talked about the forms of interference of the electrical systems in the body, and we spoke about some shielding techniques for ourselves and our families. Next we will learn how to release stored energies that are causing some stresses in our lives. One way to do this is to provide time in the morning to do some mild yoga (stretch). There are many DVDs out there that you can purchase to use in your daily regime, or now and then.

Meditation: a Powerful Tool

Meditation is often combined with yoga and is another technique that can be very powerful for stress reduction. Meditation simply means that you take a few minutes in the morning to close your eyes and focus. One way is to focus your thoughts on peaceful, happy, stress-relieving ideas. Thinking about only things that are conducive to your happiness can help realign your electrical systems by lining up your thoughts with your ultimate goals, whether you realize what they are or not. Take time to think of all the things that you have to be thankful for. Think about all of the things that you would like to see happen in your life. What are the things that will make you happy? Using this technique can be very powerful in relieving stress; not only does it relieve stress but it can actually create happiness in your life, no matter what is currently not going so well.

Music Soothes the Savage Beast

Relaxing music can help relieve stress during your stretch, meditation, or anytime you have the opportunity to listen. Certain music can help you focus mentally; this alone can help relieve stress. Being able to focus is very liberating as it helps you get a mental handle on your life and happenings by having the mental capacity to do so. This technique is very powerful for relieving stress. This is why we need to address chemical contaminations first, as they can hinder concentration as well. Music can instantly change your mood from bad to good, again being a powerful tool for stress reduction.

Prayer can be a powerful tool in stress reduction and rebalancing of the central nervous system. Prayer and meditation are not too far from the same, but prayer usually involves speaking directly to God, asking to help us on our journey. But similar to meditation, prayer can help us focus on what we have to be grateful for, what it is we truly want; it can teach us humility, which, when achieved, can ironically create pride in yourself. Not destructive pride or arrogance but a healthy respect for yourself, a good self-esteem works wonders for your ability to manage stress. When we are confident and feeling good, we open doors of opportunity that we did not know existed. Needless to say, when you can achieve your goals with confidence and ease, this creates a momentum of energy, while inertia swiftly carries you to your dreams and desires.

Needles Being Used to Open Electrical Pathways

Acupuncture is a mechanical means of opening new or reopening stifled electrical pathways within the body. It uses small needles to tap into electrical "hubs" within the body and then redirects these electrical signals where they need to go two or more electrical points. This is a very effective form of energetic rebalancing and can significantly increase the overall electrical activity within the body. As we now know, when your electrical activity is higher, it means your body is functioning as a vibrantly health body should be.

More Uses for Essential Oils

There are certain essential oils that can be used to rid the body of stored traumas and emotional issues. This can be achieved by simply using the oils with the intention and focus of relieving the body's emotional stresses. There is no need for any consultation to do this, but sometimes the added communication can be helpful. Someone who is well versed in essential oils can help with these matters. For hundreds of years, these oils were used by priests for healing of all kinds. There are still priests and other spiritual healers that can help you with these types of emotional traumas. You can utilize these oils while receiving some emotional council from a loved one or a trusted professional as well.

Need an Alignment?

Chiropractics are techniques that use mechanical manipulation of the muscles, bones, and joints. When the bones and joints are out of line, this situation can seriously interrupt electrical, lymphatic, circulatory, and digestive systems within the body. Most of the time when your bones are out of alignment, it is typically caused by a muscle pulling or pushing a bone or joint out of alignment, usually in the back or neck. When our muscles sustain injury, they tend to stiffen up. The stiffness comes from inflammation, dehydration, and contamination of the muscles. When you have severe inflammation along with electrical interference, the muscles can begin to twitch or spasm causing shooting pains.

Remove the Cause Then Realign

When the muscles are in this condition, they need to be cooled and calmed before and during the mechanical manipulation of the spinal column and neck. If these symptoms are not addressed first, the muscles will simply pull the vertebrae out of alignment again, which can cause more pain and irritation to the muscles and joints, further worsening the injury.

First we should address contamination, hydration, and rest and second a good chiropractor will often use electrical, muscular stimulation (EMS) on these injured muscles first before any manipulation techniques of the joints are implemented. Sometimes, if the injury is bad enough, a chiropractor will use only EMS for a few visits before starting the alignment process on your bones.

We all know that in our back is a spinal column; within this spinal column is our main electrical distribution center (bus). Since this is true, when the bones and joints get pulled out of place, they can seriously interrupt electrical flows, causing pain and dysfunction in the body. By realigning the bones properly, this can open new electrical pathways that have been stifled for years. This technique works not only for electrical pathway enhancement but also can open blocked circulatory, lymphatic, and other pathways in the body as well.

As these concepts found here in the book become more known and practiced, you will find over time that there are new techniques for energetic rebalancing coming out all the time. By taking time to research these things to keep up with what's new will allow you to find easier more efficient ways to achieve this balance in your life as well. Energy is one of the most misunderstood mysteries of the universe; therefore, we still have a lot to learn. The more we practice these techniques, the more we will learn on the subjects, and the more we can use this knowledge in our favor instead of against us.

E=MC2

Energy is one of the most misunderstood mysteries within our universe. According to Albert Einstein and his above-mentioned formula, all matter is made up of energy. What is energy? As far as we can tell, energy is vibration, electricity, or frequency. These terms are all synonymous with each other. The formula states that energy = matter multiplied by the square of the constant of the speed of light. This means that all matter is made of energy. Also, the formula allows us to tell how much energy is held within a mass (nuclear/atomic energy).

We Are All Made of the Same Things

Besides everything else in the world, we too are made up of matter. This matter is also made of energy, which means we and all masses are simply a vibration of energy slowed or condensed to a visible form of matter, which means we, as well as everything else we think is solid, are not solid. Because we are all made of energy, we have a frequency. This frequency we said represents electrical activity. So it seems that we are made of nothing more than the same thing that everything else is made of: energy.

If you take a look at chemistry on a molecular level, you will see that even chemical reactions are really just electrical reactions between different forms of matter (remember our water changed from H_2O to $OH-$), which is again just forms of energy combining to create new forms of energy or energy changing shape. Energy cannot be created or destroyed; it can only be changed from one form to another. This is achieved on a day-to-day basis for us. We convert matter to electricity every day; we convert food to energy in our bodies every day, and we take potential energy of all kinds and convert it to kinetic energy every day.

Energy of Many Forms

So it seems we need energy every day in order to sustain life force or electrical activity. The healthy foods that we talked about contain not only the chemical catalysts needed for function and decontamination but also contain the correct vibrations or energies that our bodies need. This fact goes overlooked as it is even more of an enigma than is the chemistry within the body.

Albert Einstein, in the early nineteenth century, proved that all matter is made of energy, and because this is true, even the things we think aren't real matter actually are, due to this fact. Even the intangible things around us that we think aren't real because they are another less lifelike or tangible form of energy are real things. This includes electricity as well as heat, microwaves, X-rays, gamma rays, light rays, and other forms of energy.

I have a customer who is a software engineer. He writes firmware for a super powerful microscope that can see down to this level of energy or vibration. These vibrations can be seen through the microscope, as they are so powerful. The vibrations exist in all matter, even when the object under the microscope is completely still. Outside vibrations, loud music, a truck driving by, a vibrating cell phone, all will affect the vibration and the way the object looks under the microscope. As a result, a dampening system was implemented as a special platform for the microscope.

Energy, Frequency, and Vibration

In the Bible (and other religious texts) it states that God "spoke" the universe into existence with his word. His words were a vibration. As we now know, vibrations are things. This is true because vibrations are energy, and all things are made of energy. This means that God is a creator of energy. He is able to wield his power of thoughts and speech to create everything in the universe. Some people know that this is true, but did you know that God gave *you* the same power only on a smaller scale.

God-Like Powers Given to Us All

We said that everything is made of energy, which includes things that are invisible or even not tangible, like electricity. We said that electricity is a vibration, well how about sound waves? They are vibrations. God turned his speech into things, which means that our speech is a creative force as well. Makes sense when you think about how sounds cause physical vibrations, which we have all experienced in some way. For example, listening to loud music and feeling it at the same time. But did you know that your thoughts are also vibrations, or because of what we now know, which is that everything is a vibration, we now know that thoughts are vibrations and therefore things!

Thomas Edison and Albert Einstein proved, with antiquated equipment of the early 1900s, that the brain is a transmitter and receiver of frequency or vibration and that all matter has a frequency and can be affected by other frequencies. Because this is true, when you think, these thoughts become things. Like attracts like, and because our thoughts are vibrations, they will attract similar vibrations, which mean that we have the power through focus to create anything we want within our life with use of the proper vibrations or in other words proper use of our thoughts and speech.

It also means that we have attracted everything in our lives that exists today, good or bad, whether we wanted it or not. Unfortunately, most people are unaware of this little-known secret, and when they do hear it, they have a hard time grasping this idea.

The Great Secret Revealed

This secret is called the law of attraction. The law of attraction is a quantum physical law that states like attracts like. The "likeness" we are talking about has specifically to do with similar frequencies. Again everything is and has a frequency; your thoughts are a frequency, and everything around you is a frequency.

This law is superior to all physical laws of the universe. We have physical laws such as gravity, which even if we don't understand how it works, still exists. But even though gravity exists we can still fly, this is due to a superior law called "lift." So even though there are physical laws of the universe, there is a hierarchy of laws. Therefore, there are quantum physical laws that exist that supersede physical laws. This is where the real magic of the universe takes place.

How Does Attraction Work in Our Lives?

How does the law of attraction apply in our lives? Simple really, when we have thoughts, whether they are good or bad, they consist of what we want or what we don't want. Our thoughts, which are vibrations, attract like vibrations into our lives. So if we are thinking about something we do not want and focusing on it most of the time, we are going to attract similar vibrations, which are things similar to what we do not want, bringing similar feelings (vibrations) to our lives. Likewise, if we are focused on what we do want most of the time, we will get exactly what we want, again by attracting the "things" (which are vibrations) that we want by putting out the frequencies of the things we desire simply by focusing on them with belief, gratitude, and passion. It takes good self esteem and self image to apply this concept, because if you don't truly believe you can have what you want or don't believe you deserve it, you won't have enough attractive powers to get what you want. You must also have enough faith that even when you can't see how you will get what you want or do what you want, you still truly believe that it will happen. It is the faith and belief in the *what* that will create and attract the *how*. The ideas come first; then how you will achieve the idea comes second (Rhonda Byrne, 2006).

We spoke of meditation as a form of energetic rebalancing. One method of meditation was to focus on what we have to be grateful for, as well as things that we would like to have or experience in our lives. By focusing on what we want continuously with enthusiasm and excitement, we continuously put out a vibration (thoughts) of the things we want in our lives, which will attract the things that will give us similar feelings.

The Secret Wasn't So Secret After All

"Ask and you shall receive," is a famous quote from the Bible, and it is absolutely true according to the law of attraction. This means that all of the things that exist in our lives right now we have attracted, because we get what we think about most of the time, even if it is not what we want! We do it by our thoughts and speech patterns. False beliefs, doubt, and fear are the main reasons we don't go for the things that we truly desire in our lives, and therefore we do not focus on them, which prevents them from coming into our lives.

Don't be upset or depressed from this! Because first off, the law of attraction says that if you are depressed, you will continue to attract depressing things, which will perpetuate your depression. Secondly, if this *is* true, then it means we can begin to rebuild our lives in a more suitable fashion immediately. We can have a life more aligned with our goals and desires. We can have anything we want if our thoughts and speech are correct and aligned with the true goals we have for our lives. Awesome!

Three Forms of God for Christians

In the Christian faith, there are described three forms of God: God the Father, the Son, and the Holy Spirit. God the Father is easy to understand because we see him as our Father or Creator. Then there is the Son of God, who was either God himself here on earth in human form, a spiritually superior human the same as the rest of us, a child of God—only closer to God than any of us have ever been, or the smartest individual who ever lived. But next there is the Holy Spirit. This concept confused me because I didn't get what other form of God this was.

Having been raised Catholic and going to Catholic schools my entire life still left me confused as to what God meant by this "Holy Spirit." Now with my understanding of energy, it makes absolute sense to me what the Holy Spirit is! The Holy Spirit is *energy!* God says that the Holy Spirit is everywhere, and that God and his Holy Spirit are inside all of us. Now that makes sense, because energy is everywhere, and it is everything, including us!

God Is a Master Scientist

God is the most incredible scientist of the universe. He has either created energy or he is simply able to wield it to his liking, and he is awesome at it! All I have to do is look around to know that this is true. God also says that he created us in his image. I think what this means is that he gave us the same power over energy that he has, only on a smaller scale. This allows us to create the things in our life that we really want by simply putting out the proper frequencies of what we want (thinking, praying). This is true but with some limitations and techniques that we will discuss.

We Can't Control Others with Strong Wills

Because we share a reality with other people in our lives, and they too have the will to create the things that they want in their lives, we cannot control everything within our lives with our thoughts, especially other people. This was not how it was meant to be anyway, since people have free will, and not even God himself chooses to control what we think or do. Therefore, we cannot control others either. This is the magic of being human! To be human in this universe is to be God-like. We have free will with the ability to create, just like God does. However, weak-willed people are easily controlled by strong-willed people.

Things Are Not the Goal

We must keep in mind that when we decide what we want, we might not know at first what the best way to achieve this goal will be, or the how, if you will. Our job is not to need a how upfront but instead to ask God for what we want, and through faith and belief in the powers God has given us, he will show us the how.

By thinking this way we open our minds to the vast possibilities of how we will achieve our goal.

Just like you know what's best for your children. Whether you realize it or not, your chief goal in life is to be blissfully happy. It is a universal goal held strong and deep within us all. If you think that you really want material things, you need to realize that they are merely catalysts to achieving the ultimate goal of happiness. That doesn't mean material things are not good; quite the opposite is true. Things can and do bring happiness, but it is important to understand that the item itself is not the goal.

We all want to be happy; it is our ultimate goal. So how do we go about becoming blissfully happy? The key is in the vibrations that you are putting out. Whatever vibrations you are emitting from your brain are attracting the matching vibrations through the law of attraction. Because we create the things in our life with our thoughts, we need to be aware of what our thoughts consist of. Don't be alarmed by this, as it is not as hard as it sounds!

Do I Have to Monitor All My Thoughts?

How do we know if our thoughts are in line with our ultimate goal? Well, how do you feel when you think about a particular dream or desire? If you feel good thinking about something, then your thoughts are in line with your ultimate bliss. If you are feeling bad when you have particular thoughts, then this is an indicator that your thoughts are not in line with your ultimate happiness. When you have inspired thought, and it makes you feel good and excited, this is an indication that you are on the right track, and action should be taken. When you have a dream or desire that you are trying to achieve, and your ideas are not exciting and joyous, then this method is not the right answer. If it *is* happy and joyous, and you are full of enthusiasm, then you are on the right track. So you see, our feelings are an invaluable tool given to us by the Father, which is to be used as an indicator of whether your thoughts are helping or hurting you.

If we can create things in our life by our thoughts, then we should see that we need to focus our thoughts on the things that we want mostly. If we constantly think of the things we don't want, whether we realize it or not, we are going to see these things manifest themselves within our lives. Why? It has to, according to the law of attraction! Any frequency or vibration that you emit from your brain will cause similar vibrations or frequencies to be attracted back to you. Any thought you have is a frequency, and it is sent from your brain, not unlike a radio transmitter, out into the universe and therefore attracts similar frequencies back to it, or back to you.

Feeling Good Now and Forever

How do you keep from feeling bad? This is not always easy and sometimes nearly impossible for some people, but the key is focusing and controlling your thoughts. We use our feelings to guide us. We need to stay positive about life and the things that are happening within it. Besides trying to keep our thoughts free from the things that will cause us to be unhappy, we need to realize that if our thoughts are in line with our goals, even "bad" stuff should make us happy. Especially at first when we begin to figure out what our dreams are and further start to focus on the things that make us feel good, we should see major changes in our lives. This is because we have begun to put the law of attraction to work for us.

What this means is that we are making changes to our lives by way of our thoughts, the worse the happening, the bigger the positive change is going to be, only if our thoughts have been aligned with our goals and good feelings. Everything happens for a reason, but it may only be a preferable reason if your thoughts and goals are clear in your mind frequently.

False Beliefs Stealing Your Future

Unfortunately, most people are very negative, and their minds and bodies are filled with freedom-stealing lies held as beliefs within their value system. Most of us walk around with a huge, negative ball of energy that craves more negative energy. This negative ball of energy is made larger through our associations with other negative people we have attracted into our lives by being unconstructive or having predominantly negative thoughts and speech patterns.

You must work hard to be successful; you must be smart to be successful; you must be in the right place at the right time in order to be successful (happy). These are all examples of lies perpetuated by the bloodsucking elite of the world in order to keep you from realizing that you too can be very successful. You can have, do, and be whatever you want if your attitude is right! Now we know that the saying "you can do anything you want when you grow up" is not just some cliché that we were taught as a child. It is real. You can do, have, and be anything you want.

The Truth Be Told: Creating New Beliefs

This is contrary to any beliefs I ever held about success. But now, with the truth revealed, I can make use of the powers that God has given me and not let doubt and fear keep me from achieving my dreams and desires. God said not to be scared, to have faith that he will take care of us, to rejoice, to sing, and dance. Why? Not only because he is our father and loves us, and like any good father wants his children to be well taken care of and happy, but because this is how we make use of the system he has put into place for our nurturing and safety.

We must rid ourselves of false beliefs in order to eliminate doubt and fear, which will allow us to have faith and go for the things that we want in our lives. This is ultimately the way that we achieve divine happiness. Believe me when I tell you that if you are miserable, know that there are many people out there who live blissfully happy lives. It *is* possible; therefore, *you too* can be blissfully happy!

Spiritual Guidelines from the Past

If we are happy and feeling good all the time, then we are not experiencing any fear, worry, anger, resentment, envy, jealousy, hatred, etc. Notice anything about some of the terminology used here? Some of these are cardinal sins. Sins to me are simply guidelines to follow in order to lead a happy healthy life, not rules put in place by an oppressive God to control us. These were used to control us not by God but by other men through history. They were using these concepts to wield their power under the guise of divine law.

If we follow the guidelines and avoid these feelings, we can eventually experience heaven in our lives here on earth; not to mention you'll feel better immediately. If we don't follow the guidelines for how to use the system, the system still exists, and it will work against us! This is not what God has in store for you! He did not leave you here to fend for yourself, instead he left behind his tools and resources for you to use. We are able to create all the things in life we want, to be anything we want, and to be happy!

Doesn't that sound like what you would want for your children? You wouldn't go away for vacation and leave young children alone to take care of themselves without making sure they were going to be okay and be provided with everything they need, would you? Your heavenly Father wouldn't do that to you either. You just need to have faith that this is true!

Skeptics Can See the Logic

If you're having a hard time with the law of attraction, you should still agree that if we focus on everything that is good in our lives, it trains us to look for all the good possibilities that the world has to offer, which is where luck, opportunity, and those things come from. If we only focus on the lack, not only do we push away the possibilities for happiness, by way of vibration, but we refuse to see them when they do appear, regardless of how or why we think they manifested in the first place.

"If you think you can or you can't, either way you are right," Henry Ford once said. This statement is not only true due to the law of attraction, but it is true in the sense that if we decide we cannot do something based on our current situation and belief system, even when our circumstances do change, we won't have the eyes to see it. We still have this idea that we are still not able to do it. This leads to the lack of awareness in the existence of the all the things we need to achieve our goal, even when these resources are right in front of our noses.

We Live in a Shared Reality of Energy

Keep in mind, in order to be in the right place at the right time and to seize opportunity when it presents itself, you will have to take some action. One cannot create things in their lives without doing anything. This concept is ridiculous. Meditation alone does not create success unless your goal is genuinely to be the greatest at meditation. We need to consider this concept and go live our lives with a renewed passion. Stay focused on what's positive in your life, so when the law of attraction presents itself with the opportunity of a lifetime, you'll be there to seize the moment.

So you can see it is imperative for us to get a handle on our health and to gain clarity of mind, so we can clearly decide what are our dreams and desires in this life will be. Furthermore, we need to get a handle on our thoughts in order to begin to create the life we have always wanted, first with our thoughts, and later our actions. This is exactly what God has intended for you and the life God wants for you! God wants you to be happy. How you go about that is *your* decision.

Using the Law of Attraction

To summarize, in order to put the law of attraction to work for you, here are the basic steps: First, declare exactly what it is you want. Be very specific and thorough. Write down everything that you want to do have or be in your life. While you do this, let there be no limitations to your dreams and desires. Write as if there are no limitations to what you can do, have, and be. Don't let time, money, education, or good looks stop you from going for it! Update this list by adding and subtracting things as your desires change. Don't worry about how you are going to achieve these things.

Meditate for a few minutes daily on these concepts. This way you will be focused on them and begin to come up with a game plan as where to start and how to do it. Always remember, we need to use our feelings to guide our decisions. If we are excited and enthusiastic about the idea of the action and felt good just performing the action, then we know we are on the right track. If we feel anxious, uncomfortable, scared, etc., then we are not choosing the correct path or means to get us where we want to go. This brings us to step two.

Faith Makes All Things Possible

Believe that you can achieve all your dreams and desires. Get excited about the new powers you have harnessed and how they are going to help bring you everything you want. Act and feel as close to already having achieved these things as possible. Frequently visualize yourself having already achieved your desires. Make a vision board of pictures, text, audio, and video that contain the things that you would like to manifest into your life. Tenacity and determination are the results of faith and belief. When you believe you can, you won't give up!

Be Thankful and Live in a State of Gratitude

Third, remember all the things in your life that you already have to be happy and grateful for. Reflect on this several times a day. Even if you see your life as really dreadful, I guarantee with the right outlook you will see that there are plenty of things in your life to be grateful for. This will (or should) improve your mood if you are feeling bad. When we look at all the resources that we have available to us, it keeps us open to the possibility of more unrealized resources. This is what it means to be in the right place at the right time or to be lucky.

You Must Take Action when Opportunity Knocks

Fourth, take action! When opportunity or inspired thoughts come into your life, thoughts that make you feel really good and excited, these are the means of the law of attraction trying to deliver you to your ultimate goal. This is where belief and faith come into play. If you don't believe you can, then you won't, even when the opportunity is available to you. Doubt and fear or a lack of faith will keep us from taking action. These are actions that could be wonderful, life-changing rides, skyrocketing you to your chosen destiny. We must have faith in ourselves and our inner strength in order to take action. So I ask you, what will you do with your inner powers?

Starting to Think Differently

Well, if you've made it this far, I'm thinking you either really like to read, you're starting to think a little differently, or both! Maybe these concepts were only reinforced for you, and you've known about them all along. Maybe this information somehow seems so familiar, even though you've never actually read or heard anything like it before. This is how I felt when I was first introduced to this information.

Information Passed on to You

Remember that I am not a doctor of any kind. I am just the messenger here. I did not invent any of the concepts in the book, other than what I specifically stated was my opinion. My opinions are formed through the internalization of the information, through research and mindset, and finally application with successful results, which is why I believe so strongly in these concepts. Although I try to remain teachable and open-minded, I will never waver from my beliefs and trust in God and the truly all natural.

Always Consult Your Licensed Health Practitioner

You should always consult your doctor before doing any diet or exercise program. Always use licensed professionals for all of your alternative healthy techniques. If you have a disease and are taking medicine of any kind, this is especially true because of possible interaction problems we talked about earlier in the book. If you take medicines of *any* kind, you need to be aware of possible interactions between this drug and all other substances, including vegetables, herbs, supplements, as well as herbicides, pesticides, artificial flavors and colors, and other chemicals that we expose ourselves to every day.

Lots of Information and Controversy

Obviously the information contained in this book is somewhat controversial and vast in category and volume. This is only the basics, just a bird's eye view of what is actually going on. As we move into the future, there will be more information to keep up with. Again, if you have the right mindset and awareness, it's pretty easy to figure out whether a product is safe or a concept is correct. If you get informed, you will adapt the ability to see through the lies, especially in the media. Hopefully if I haven't given you new eyes, I have at least planted the seeds for new ones, which I'm hoping you'll cultivate and develop on your own. Always remember the concept that if it is new to the body, has not existed or been used by the body throughout evolution, or not made *for* the body by the Creator, it is potentially dangerous to our health, and we should not expose ourselves to it in any way!

Come and Join Our Health Club Community

If you like what you have read here and want to learn more you can visit my website at www.CleanRegimeHealthCoaching.com where we have much more information for your use. Also, I offer online health coaching and education. I have all of the products you read about available, including the actual products that I use or have used as tools for achieving vibrant health. Some products I will offer directly to you, and I can show you how to get others. The website is loaded with diet plans, meal plans, recipes, more health tips, and information on how to find safe food, hygiene, and cleansing products. Blog about your health tips and techniques and hear about what others are doing to stay healthy. Continue to learn more about how we can live a spiritually uplifting and healthy lifestyle together.

With Cleansing Comes Clarity and Awakenings

I have spoken to several people who know some of the topics covered in this book and who have tried some different cleansing techniques. These people have had similar experiences to mine, where they state they feel younger and that it has even been an awakening, due to the clarity of mind that was gained. This is always awesome to hear, because it confirms all I believe about how to achieve vibrant health. We can't forget that our brains are organs that need energy and sustenance in order to function properly. When our bodies are running optimally, we can begin to gain spiritual awareness of ourselves and the world around us. Without our minds, we have no control over our thoughts and therefore no control over our destiny, ourselves, or our happiness.

Remember and Master the Basics

The concepts found in these pages are the foundational basics to maintaining our health. We must understand these concepts as they have everything to do with achieving vibrant health. Let's take a look at some real-life stories consisting of a few examples of how poor attitude, lack of education, and improper diet can cause tragedy in people's lives. Remember that I care about you and others. I want to help you help yourselves, but it takes change (action) on your part. Here are some examples that might explain why.

Sad Story with a Lesson to Learn

"Sally," who is a friend of a friend, has a hard time believing or even listening to me about any of the concepts contained here in the book. The resistance is mostly about her diet consisting of junk and processed foods. This friend of mine rarely says anything to people about these concepts unless she feels compelled to, which is a rare occasion because she knows how angry and offensive people get when talking about this stuff. However, she does consistently speak to Sally about it, mostly because she complains about weight and health problems on a consistent basis (law of attraction: focusing on what you don't want or have). About a year or so ago, this friend's spouse had a heart attack!

Naturally I became more concerned about Sally and her spouse, so my friend began to speak to and offer information about how to eat right and so forth. As usual, Sally didn't listen. They wouldn't fight about it, but my friend would typically be stifled fairly quickly by Sally to stop talking about it. I care about family and friends, so I felt really bad when I found out about the heart attack. I knew I could help with nutrition and other concepts, but I was stifled and unable to because they didn't want to listen.

This is why I get so frustrated when people don't listen to reason and later start to, or continue to have worsening complaints of health problems, most likely caused by doing exactly what I tried to tell them to avoid. There are no definitive answers to what caused this heart attack, but some of the lifestyle choices being made on a regular basis by this couple were definitely suspect. I also know deep down that attitude and stress management, are huge factors, and must be considered when trying to decide; what are the dangers to our health that are hidden within our not so clean regime?

Sally tends to be a proud, bitter, unhappy, poor soul, which is why she and I clash, I think. The point here is that she is always negative and complaining. This is a reflection of how unhappy that she is on the inside with her life and the way it is going. She doesn't realize that in order to be happy, you must focus on happy things, which then leads to the attraction of more happy things. This creates more happy feelings and so forth. With a simple shift in her awareness, she could turn her life around seemingly instantly. Sally looks up to my friend and has listened from time to time with an open mind but still has not made the changes that are needed to improve her quality of life. I am sure my friend has been able to reach and teach Sally plenty over the years; however, not much has changed in the couple's unhealthy regime.

Not a few months later, I was shocked to hear more bad news from this couple. Sally was diagnosed with breast cancer. Needless to say, I was devastated to hear this, as I wished only the best of health and happiness to all people, especially family and friends. Naturally I wanted to help with some advice, again on diet and nutrition. My friend was definitely not trying to play doctor, and as always, I instruct everyone to consult a licensed healthcare provider before changing anything in their regime, but I tried to offer some advice on what to avoid as a cancer patient.

And, of course, I got the same result: Sally didn't want to hear it. She went to the doctor for the conventional treatment, without any regard for additional or alternative therapies. She continued to live an unhealthy lifestyle, regardless of disease manifesting itself. Close minded and bitter, basically paralyzed by a negative attitude, she was unable to change anything. Naturally having such a serious health problem can devastate us and our family, but this way of thinking is, in my opinion, only going to make things worse, regardless of any additional or alternative therapies. As much as it kills me, I can't do anything to help. Sally is definitely not going to listen to me, especially if she doesn't listen to her best friend.

More recently I found out that Sally went to see a surgeon to have both her breasts removed. I guess this is pretty common today, which is why you see so much "for the cure" stuff going on today. It just seems to get worse as time goes on. Hopefully Sally can turn her life around and make some positive changes starting with open mindedness. Sad story, but it's true. Here is another real-life story.

Living with a Poor Diet and Attitude

Growing up I met some friends that I will call the Smiths. The Smiths were a family of three boys, a mom, and a dad. Although we were friends, I realized that they were all very negative in their outlook from the beginning. The father was successful in education and finance, and he had a good job, which brought a good salary. Despite this fact, they were all very depressed, negative, and unhappy in general. Now it is important to mention that these people also had a very poor diet, one that I would consider to be about as bad as it gets, except for eating only fast food, although there was a lot of that being consumed as well. This might not have been uncommon among families at the time, but not for me. I was blessed with a mother who understood what eating right meant.

Early on, soon after we became friends, Mrs. Smith was diagnosed with and later died from cancer. I can remember her wearing the bandana to cover her balding head. This was back in the 1980s, so you can imagine that chemotherapy was a lot harder on the body back then. We were all very sad for the rest of the family, and we were all there to offer support for them.

Soon after, one of the boys was diagnosed with cancer as well. Fortunately he went into remission, and his life was spared. As kids, we were scared, but our friend never left us, so we were okay. During our late teenage years, one of the brothers took recreational use of alcohol a bit too far and later embarked on a lifelong journey of alcoholism and, worse still, heroin use. I have since heard stories of rehabilitation and relapse over the years, but as far as I know he is still alive and an addict.

Now the first brother who had cancer later was able to survive a near-fatal car accident, where he lost one of his semi-vital organs. Incredibly to us, as he was but a frail young lad who previously had cancer, he made it through. We were all relieved. Ironically, this particular brother was the jolliest of them all, so I have to give him credit on joy and passion; however, he did lack any real "vision" or any tenacity to achieve his dreams.

Now the third brother was probably the most intelligent one of them all. He had the most promise in my mind as to being the sibling who would do the most with his life. However, this gentleman (God rest his soul) was not immune to the negativity and poor diet within the family milieu. Despite his intelligence, he showed no interest in the high-tech education and career of his father, which was displayed all over their house, which I found intriguing and compelling. Regardless of this fact, I still saw the most promise from him.

At the end of his teenage life, just as the boy was entering into manhood, he was struck down with a broken back from a tragic accident. This unfortunate event landed him in a wheelchair for life, with metal rods in his back and ongoing pain. At this point he and most of the people caring for him believed he was "all done." Because of the accident, he wouldn't be able to do anything with his life. Although his existence touched the lives of his friends, which was a beautiful gift that I was blessed with, he did not seem to achieve many of his dreams or desires beyond the accident.

Because of the pain from the back injury and reconstructive surgeries that had to be redone because they were done incorrectly the first time, he was introduced to a life of conventional pain management with the use of opiates. Naturally, over time these drugs didn't work anymore, as he developed a tolerance and addiction to these drugs. He then, through the association with "others" that used it, began to make use of heroin as well. This friend is no longer with us, as he has recently died with complications connected with being a paraplegic and bedridden, and as we know, a *very* poor diet and attitude.

Mr. Smith, as we can imagine, was devastated by the loss of his wife and mother of his children, as well as the other stressful accidents and situations taking place in their lives. For years I would comment on the fact that he still doesn't have any love in his life. I believed that his fallen wife would want him to find love in this physical world in order to help him live a fulfilling life beyond the one they shared. And although he and I shared some of the same passions, to me he was still a solemn soul, very quiet, and often angry. As far as I know he is still alone, now dealing with the loss of his son as well.

A More Personal Story

My last story is about my own father. He was a man with a very poor self-image. He was very proud and grew up in the nineteen thirties. I knew his dad only until I was six, as he later died. However, I was told by my older siblings, also related to my grandfather on this side, that he was a tough character, always dysfunctional and abusive. I later realized that, coupled with the life-altering trauma of fighting in WWII, these facts were the root of my father's emotional problems and insecurities.

Unfortunately, unlike a lot of immigrant families who held onto a healthier lifestyle more closely related to their heritage, my dad did not carry any of these heirlooms, especially within the realm of nutrition or healthy lifestyle. As most of the soldiers of the past and present, my father turned to alcohol and drugs as a means of coping with his emotional pain. This lifestyle continued until he reached the point where his health problems caused him to need too much medicine and therefore; he could no longer enjoy a drink.

Fortunately, my mother and father got married and created me, and I love this gift of life that they facilitated through the power of our Creator. Unfortunately their union did not last, as my mother and father are two completely different people. This ended in about six years. Due to a lack of open-mindedness, my father never seemed to learn any techniques to remedy his relationship, nor did he ever seem to identify with any of his problems with feelings, emotions, and resulting destruction of relationships with his friends and family. Some of my family still do not speak with him, as he can be a disaster to others in certain situations.

While my parents were together, my father enjoyed the luxury of having quality food prepared for him daily by my mom. As I mentioned, she understood what a well-balanced meal consisted of and what quality food was. When they split up, these concepts didn't seem to stick, because he didn't seem to mind when his diet drastically changed after the divorce. His new wife, my stepmom, although very loving and loyal, does not know how to take care of herself properly, as far as health is concerned, and therefore cannot take care of my father properly either, although she has spent most of her life trying.

As a result, my father has led an increasingly deteriorating lifestyle, which has robbed him of his wealth and golden years. Because of the lack of education, spiritual inspiration, and proper diet, and the fact that the two of them are very negative, neither one of them having fulfilled their dreams and desires (like most people) because of having to deal with all the woes and health problems that they share and focus on. And even though they have a wealth of resources at their disposal, they choose to go through life feeling victimized and powerless, doing whatever everyone else does or tells them to do.

Though I continuously prove myself to be knowledgeable and correct about being healthy, eating well, and avoiding negative behavior, he still won't listen to my advice when he doesn't have to or want to. As a result he and his wife have and continue to live with compounding health problems.

I'm forced to sit and watch the two of them continue to deteriorate and be further victimized by corporate greed, all the while getting continuously worse. Every time I talk to them it's a new story of woe and misery, combined with some crazy idea of hope as to how they are going to remedy it with more pills. I get so overwhelmingly furious but have learned to hold my tongue, as it has done no good thus far.

Writing it down in a book hopefully detaches the reader from the emotional confrontation involved with discussing these controversial ideas with me about how to be truly healthy and stay that way, and it also hopefully gives them a chance to internalize the information more easily by reading, rather than through short emotional confrontations. However, he still shows no interest, as he has the belief that it is too farfetched and he cannot understand it anyway, based on the confusion he experiences as a result of listening to the things I continue to say on a regular basis.

Learn from Other People's Successes and Mistakes

We have all heard of mentoring. This is how skills are handed down to the apprentice from the master. Success does rub off! This is without question a true statement, maybe not for all of us, but for those of us who learn from observation or the teaching of others who have achieved successes, in order to figure out how to achieve the same successes for ourselves.

The same is true in the opposite direction. If we see, or more importantly don't see someone who has what we want, and we stay close-minded to the techniques used to achieve these successes, then we will never succeed at getting what we want. We too are trying to reinvent the wheel and probably won't achieve what we really wanted in the first place. This is especially tragic when a loved one or friend is having problems, and you are trying to help them because you have experience and success with that vey same issue, but the person still is unable to see the reality of what is being shown to them.

I don't want this to be you! Maybe there are evil people out there who do, but I don't earn a living off of other people's misery and hardships. I'm in the business of enhancing people's lives, trying to help them figure out what is right for *their* health and happiness as a health coach.

There Is a Place for All Forms of Medicine

Despite the bashing that I have given the world of unnatural products, like drugs, you must remember that if you are diagnosed with a life-threatening disease, you need to use all of the resources available to you, including drugs and surgery. Obviously, lives are being saved every day with some of the new technologies in the world of conventional medicine, but it is so profitable that it is extremely overused. You need to instead learn how to increase the odds that you will not need this type of therapy. But again, you cannot completely eliminate the need for this type of medicine, as you cannot control everything that happens to you, including injury from falls and other types of accidents.

Please take into consideration the things I've talked about in this book, as I believe it will help you live the spiritually rewarding and vibrantly healthy lifestyle, which myself and my family enjoy every day. I wish nothing but for God to bless you on your journey to vibrant health. Remember I am here to assist you on your way with answers to your questions about health as you go along.

Always remember to live, laugh, and love often! Consider daily the things that you should be grateful for. Learn what feeling grateful is about. Do this by identifying your blessings and by helping others. When we see others appreciate us, we learn what it looks like, and we can begin to see and feel what true gratitude feels like in us.

Never forget if your health is not up to par and your body is not functioning properly, it becomes impossible to awaken your inner powers. Without utilizing proper maintenance techniques for our bodies, not unlike a formula racecar, our bodies cannot perform and stay in the race. Learn what types of methods and tools work for you in your "healthy pit stop," and use them on a regular basis. Don't be afraid to treat yourself to some of your favorite junk foods now and then, but only if you have your body chemistry and overall health under control first—if it isn't already. This way you won't become overwhelmed with contamination. Good luck! God bless you all!

References

ASCE, "Drinking Water". http://www.infrastructurereportcard. org/fact-sheet/drinking-water 6-19-2012

Byrne, Rhonda. *The Secret*, DVD. Ts Production LLC. Orlando, FL. 2006

Cohen, Robert. "Milk the Deadly Poison". Argus Publishing 1997

Cuomo, Chris. ABC News. "New Studies Find Yaz More Risky Than Other Leading Birth Control Pills: ABC News Investigates"- Oct 14, 2011. http://abcnews.go.com/TheLaw/studies-find-yaz-risky-leading-birth-control-pills/story?id=14741760 6-19-2012

Deyanda Flint. "The Effects of Herbicides & Pesticides on Humans". eHow. Com.

http://www.ehow.com/facts_5636303_effects-herbicides-pesticides-humans.html 6-19-2012

Enagic USA. "What is Kangen Water®?" http://www.enagic. com/watertheory.php. 6-19-2012

Hill, Napoleon. "Think and Grow Rich". Success Co. Books: Lexington, KY. 2009

Ian Blair Hamilton. "Alkaline Water & ORP Explained. Or is a 20 Minute Read Worth an Extra 5 Years of Life?" IonLife, Australia http://www.ionizers.org/alkaline-water.html. 6-19-2012

John Hopkins. "Johns Hopkins researchers solve mystery of Warburg effect" -2011 http://www.news-medical.net/news/20110602/Johns-Hopkins-researchers-solve-mystery-of-Warburg-effect.aspx. 6-19-2012

Kenner, Robert *Food Inc.*, DVD, Participant Media, 2008

Librarian50, "Why is health care in America so bad compared with other countries?"

Askville by Amazon, http://askville.amazon.com/health-care-America-compared-countries/AnswerViewer.do?requestId=12175921. 6-19-2012

"What is Kobe Beef?". http://www.askthemeatman.com/kobe_beef.htm. 6-19-2012

Moore, Michael. *Capitalism a Love Story*, DVD, Dog Eat Dog Films, 2009

Osmunson, DDS, Dr. Bill. "Professional Perspectives: Fluoride in Tap Water". YouTube.com. http://www.youtube.com/watch?v=_Ys9q1cvKGk. 6-19-2012

Stewart, David. "Healing Oils of the Bible". Life Science Publishers: Orem, Utah. 2009

Sustainable Table. "The Issues; Additives" http://www.sustainabletable.org/issues/additives/ 6-19-2012

Trading Corp, US Niagara. "Import of Active Pharmaceutical Ingredients".

http://www.usniagaratrading.com/services.html 6-19-2012

Trudeau, Kevin. "Natural cures 'they' don't want you to know about". Alliance Publishing Group. Birmingham, AL 2005

Trudeau, Kevin. "Your Wish Is Your Command". Alliance Publishing Group. Birmingham, AL 2004

Trudeau, Kevin. "Your Wish Is Your Command" CD Set. Global Information Network, 2009

Tuberose.com, "Fluoride". http://www.tuberose.com/Fluoride.html. 6-19-2012

Vassey, Christopher. "The Acid-Alkaline Diet for optimum health". Healing Arts Press Rochester, VT. 2006

Watson, Molly. *About.com*. "What Is Cage-Free Chicken?"

http://localfoods.about.com/od/localfoodsglossary/g/What-Are-Cage-Free-Chicken.htm 6-19-2012

Koch, Wendy. "WHO: Air pollution kills more than 2 million annually".-Sep 26, 2011 USA TODAY, http://content.usa-today.com/communities/greenhouse/post/2011/09/who-air-pollution-causes-more-than-two-million-annual-deaths-/1. 6-19-2012

Wulffson, MD, Robin. "Antiperspirants and deodorants linked to breast cancer".–January 26, 2012

http://www.emaxhealth.com/11306/antiperspirants-and-deodorants-linked-breast-cancer 6-19-2012

About the Author

In late fall 2010, I began to write the very first manuscript of my life. It seems so overwhelmingly impossible to actually write down in an organized fashion all of the thoughts that I have crammed in my head, and which I hoped to share with you. However, I have been compelled to do so, and so this begins my first journey as an author. Thanks for reading my book! I was forty years old when I began to write this book and further spent a few years trying to perfect it for you. Today I am forty-two going on thirty, at least with how I feel and how I look. I grew up and currently reside in a larger New Hampshire town along the Massachusetts border. I am a tradesman by profession, or more specifically a plumbing, heating, and cooling contractor. However, contemplating, pondering, researching, and reacting to the wonders of nature are nothing new for me.

I graduated from high school and later attended some college (associates CIT program) but hold no degree. I went to trade school, and I am a licensed professional. I have an IQ of around 140, based on a few different tests that I have taken over the years. I love science and nature, and to me there is no way to separate the two, as our Creator is the most genius scientist. I have always been interested in health and fitness, as this entails the science of the body.

I have been working out and watching my diet for around twenty-five years or more. I am always eager to find out more information on nutrition, health, the human body, and its functions. Because our Creator has given me this incredible, biological vehicle, I feel it's my duty to learn how to take care of it. This is the only way that I will have the ability to properly maintain this high-tech car of mine so I will be able to achieve all the dreams and desires of my life at lightning speed.

Please remember that I did not invent any of the concepts in this book. My intelligence and profession allows me only to read, understand, and implement this information, which has been figured out by scientists and or other people who are smarter than I am or by people who have made it their life's work to solve these mysteries. All of the information contained in this book can be found in other books and on the Internet. My only hope is that this book finds you well and leaves you spiritually uplifted and enlightened, so that *you too* will be able to achieve and maintain vibrant health for yourself and your family.